Studies in Disorders of Communication

General Editors:

Professor David Crystal
Honorary Professor of Linguistics, University College of North Wales,
Bangor

Professor Ruth Lesser
University of Newcastle upon Tyne

Professor Margaret Snowling
University of Newcastle upon Tyne

Communication and Adults with Learning Disabilities

New Map of An Old Country

Anna van der Gaag and Klara Dormandy

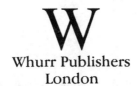

Whurr Publishers
London

© 1993 Whurr Publishers Ltd
19B Compton Terrace, London N1 2UN, England

Reprinted 1994

British Library Cataloguing-in-Publication Data
A catalogue record for this book is available from the
British Library

ISBN 1-870332-27-X

Printed and bound in the UK by Athenaeum Press Ltd, Gateshead, Tyne & Wear.

Preface

> The end of all our exploring
> Will be to arrive at where we started
> And know the place for the first time.

T.S. Eliot
The Four Quartets
(Little Gidding)

There are no new ideas in the world, only different ways of looking at it. This book is a contribution to that process. It is a book about communication and learning disabilities in adults, written for professionals and carers with a particular focus on the contribution of the speech and language therapist.

The main aim of the book is to explore connections between ideas and concepts from related fields and to put them into the context of learning disabilities. Some chapters have been written for those new to working with adults, others will serve to reinforce and affirm ideas that have already been put to use by practitioners. It is in this sense that the book is a new map of an old country. As its authors we serve as map makers, attempting to highlight those streets and buildings that have previously gone unnoticed or that no-one has believed to be there at all.

This work has emerged from ongoing teaching and research into the nature of communication on the one hand and an exploration of clinical practice issues in relation to learning disabilities on the other.

Anna van der Gaag
Klara Dormandy
February 1993

Acknowledgements

Many people have contributed to this book, some through debates and discussions, others by quite specific information and ideas that are disseminated through these pages, and still others by believing that it could be written. A number of individuals deserve special mention: Phil Davies, specifically for his contribution to Chapter 9 and more generally for his encouragement and his collaboration, Peter Mudford for his helpful comments on earlier drafts of Chapter 1 and Alison Kidd for contributing her expertise as well as her support. Thanks also go to Marilyn Goulding, Vicky Baker, Sue Whitefoot, Liz Tuck, Diane Webb, Marion Sculthorpe, Elizabeth Bridgman, Marina Sloan, Lucy Hurst Brown, Alison Keens, Tessa Smith, Alex Hitchins and Briege McLean and to the staff and clients at The Royal Forest Centre and at Fairtide.

The contribution of those who took part in the workshops on defining professional competence is also gratefully acknowledged.

We would also like to thank the three anonymous referees for their comments and very helpful suggestions.

Finally, our thanks go Davie and to John, without whose quiet support and good humour this book could never have been written.

General preface

This series focuses upon disorders of speech language and communication, bringing together the techniques of analysis, assessment and treatment which are pertinent to the area. It aims to cover cognitive, linguistic, social and education aspects of language disability, and therefore has relevance within a number of disciplines. These include speech therapy, the education of children and adults with special needs, teachers of the deaf, teachers of English as a second language and of foreign languages, and educational and clinical psychology. The research and clinical findings from these various areas can usefully inform one another and, therefore, we hope one of the main functions of this series will be to put people within one profession in touch with developments in another. Thus, it is our editorial policy to ask authors to consider the implications of their findings for professions outside their own and for fields with which they have not been primarily concerned. We hope to engender an integrated approach to theory and practice and to produce a much-needed emphasis on the description and analysis of language as such, as well as on the provision of specific techniques of therapy, remediation and rehabilitation

Whilst it has been our aim to restrict the series to the study of language disability, its scope goes considerably beyond this. Many previously neglected topics have been included where these seem to benefit from contemporary research in linguistics, psychology, medicine, sociology, education and English studies. Each volume puts its subject matter in perspective and provides an introductory slant to its presentation. In this way we hope to provide specialised studies which can be used as texts for components of teaching courses at undergraduate and postgraduate levels, as well as material directly applicable to the needs of professional workers.

David Crystal
Ruth Lesser
Margaret Snowling

Contents

Part I
Current Issues in
Assessment

Chapter 1
Introduction

According to William Whewell, 'There is a mask of theory over the whole face of nature' (Whewell, 1847). Everything we look at we see from our own particular perspective, with certain prejudices arrived at through our experience and training. This is as true for speech and language therapists as it is for any other group of individuals. Speech and language therapists look at the world in certain ways, and their working practice is determined as much by their beliefs and values as by their techniques and training.

There are a number of precepts which have influenced speech and language therapy's working practice in quite fundamental ways. The first is that speech and language therapy is partly a scientific endeavour, based upon scientific principles and practices. This means that it strives towards objectivity, measurability, quantification and cause and effect explanations of human communicative behaviour. A second relates to the various paradigm shifts that influence not only how a therapist might view the world but also how she will work with her clients.

Is Speech and Language Therapy a Science?

This book would suggest that such precepts have led to a number of misconceptions about the theory and practice of therapy, and about the relationship between speech and language therapy and 'science'. Is speech and language therapy a science? Is science what defines speech and language therapy? Medawar (1982) gave the following definition of scientific endeavour which may shed some light on the subject.

> The purpose of scientific enquiry is not to compile an inventory of factual information...it must begin with a story about a possible world – a story which we invent and criticise and modify as we go along so that it ends by being, as nearly as we can make it, a story about real life (p.111).

Speech and language therapists should perhaps see themselves as storytellers, not merely list writers. By and large, they probably do. But perhaps they sometimes lack appropriate models upon which to base their practice. They know what to do, but do not necessarily have the epistemological basis they would like to have for doing it.

This may well be because they start out with false assumptions about themselves and their discipline. They perceive themselves as speech scientists, with the emphasis on scientist, when in fact they will never be scientists in the same sense of the word as biologists or mathematicians or chemists.

Bench (1989) argues very convincingly that speech and language therapy, a relatively young discipline, should not even aspire to becoming a (natural) science. It is driven as much by the humanities and social sciences as it is by the natural sciences, and yet it seeks to identify with natural science over and above the other two. One of the defining features of a natural science is that it has a core paradigm upon which all existing knowledge and the search for new knowledge are based (Kuhn, 1970). Bench (1989) suggests that speech and language therapy will never have a core paradigm in the way that biology or zoology have because it cannot have a consensual body of knowledge. Rather, it is made up of a whole series of different types of knowledge and different paradigms that are quite distinct. For example, the knowledge required to work with an adult with a voice problem will be very different from the knowledge required to work with a child with autism. For the first one knowledge of the anatomy and physiology of the larynx is essential, whereas such knowledge would not be essential for the second. This 'catholicism', as Bench calls it, precludes the development of a core paradigm.

Bench's observations are borne out by a recent study of the professional competence of speech and language therapists working with three distinct groups of people with communication difficulties: the elderly and adults with acquired neurological disorders, children with developmental delays and people with learning disabilities (Davies and van der Gaag, 1992a,b; van der Gaag and Davies, 1992a,b). This study showed how a group of 67 speech and language therapy experts working in these three specialties identified relatively few consensus items of knowledge across all three specialties. A further 657 therapists throughout the UK were then asked to agree or disagree with the list of consensus items identified by the 67 'experts'.There was a strong consensus of agreement on the knowledge base within each specialty, but there was very little overlap between the three. This finding would support Bench's view that speech and language therapy does not have a core paradigm, but a number of paradigms which coexist and direct different branches of the discipline.

If speech and language therapy is content to accept that it has no core paradigm, then perhaps it will deal more constructively with the differences that exist between its different branches. Speech and language therapists who work with adults with learning disabilities have for some time recognised that there are considerable differences between their own practices and those of their colleagues in other areas. This we would argue is because the epistemological basis of speech and language therapy varies depending upon the specialty in which therapists work. Speech and language therapists working with people with learning disabilities are, quite rightly, influenced by the theories and philosophies that govern the learning disabilities field as well as by those within speech and language therapy. These theories and philosophies are drawn from a wide range of disciplines, not all of which would even wish to consider themselves 'scientific'.

This brings us to another interesting question: in what sense do speech and language therapists consider themselves as 'artists' as well as 'scientists'?

Some practitioners have difficulty accepting that the practice of therapy is first and foremost a creative and imaginative process, because in some strange way it will detract from the status of the speech therapist as a 'speech scientist'. This is because creativity and imagination are traditionally associated with the more obviously creative professionals, such as painters, musicians and writers, but not with speech and language therapists. What Medawar (1982) and others have argued is that the creative process is present in 'scientific' as well as 'artistic' pursuits. One of the misconceptions of 'science' is that it exists, by definition, in opposition with 'art'. Art is associated with creativity, inventiveness, freedom of ideas, absence of boundaries. In contrast, science is often associated with a deterministic view of the world, of cause and effect relationships, of rules. This polarity exists more in the mind than in the practice of either art or science.

Medawar (1982) suggests that imaginative and creative processes are at the heart of what scientists do. Science is indeed about quantification and measurability, but it is not only about these. Not all scientific thought or action is propelled by logic alone. Behind every hypothesis there is an idea that is subsequently subjected to rigorous and systematic investigation, often using a predetermined structure. This is true for artists who paint or write songs. They will have an idea which must then be developed in the context of certain medium-specific principles. For example, the rules of music will constrain the way in which the musician formulates his phrases. This is equally true for the speech and language therapist, who formulates a hypothesis and then explores it using speech and language therapy principles and techniques.

Do speech and language therapists see themselves and their work in this light? Do they perceive themselves as being creative when they decide on a particular course of action using particular methods and materials? Certainly, their perception of themselves will have an influence on the way they work with clients. If being a 'scientist' means thinking and acting creatively in the context of a therapeutic relationship, formulating hypotheses and experimenting in a systematic way, then it should be a framework that speech and language therapists endorse wholeheartedly. However, if being a scientist places boundaries upon the process of intervention so that creativity and experimentation become stifled, then 'scientist' is not a label to aspire to.

The Shifting Paradigms of Science and Speech and Language Therapy

The history of science is characterised by continuous change. This can be triggered by new knowledge or new ways of looking at the world. As Pickering (1987) pointed out, there is more than one approach to knowing, whatever your subject. There is, or should be, a constant growth both in how to know and what to know. Kuhn (1970) observed that scientists frequently adopt a new theory and discard an old one because they become more interested in the problems that can be explored with the new one. It must also be acknowledged, however, that new theories are not always an improvement on old ones. As Planck (1949) said: ' a new scientific truth does not triumph by convincing its opponents and making them see light, but rather because its opponents eventually die, and a new generation grows up that is familiar with it'. Some examples of this are given below.

From classical physics to quantum physics

The most obvious example of such a paradigm shift in scientific theory is the change from what has been called the classical or Newtonian world view of physics to the radical alternative put forward by quantum theorists such as Planck (1900), and Heisenberg (1926). The Newtonian view sees and studies the world as deterministic and mechanistic, where everything can be explained in terms of cause and effect or, in other words, linear relationships. According to this theory, there will ultimately be a set of laws that allow scientists to predict everything that goes on in the world. In contrast, quantum theories do not allow a single definite outcome from any action. As Hawking explains: 'It [quantum theory] predicts a number of different possible outcomes, which brings an unavoidable element of unpredictability or randomness into science' (Hawking, 1988). Quantum theories assert that phenomena have no meaning in isolation and should therefore not be studied in isolation. They also assert that there is a subjective element in every scientific observation – one can never be entirely objective.

Quantum theory has probably been responsible for one of the most dramatic paradigm shifts in modern scientific thought .

Chaos theory is a more recent example of quantum theory which has been popularised by authors such as Glieck (1987). Chaos theorists suggest that the world is determined as much by irregularity as by regularity, as much by chaos as by order. According to Glieck, chaos theory has influenced almost every field of the so-called 'hard' sciences: mathematics, chemistry, physics, biology, ecology, epidemiology (Lorenz, 1963; Wolf; 1983, Huberman and Hogg, 1984; Miles, 1984; Ford, 1985; Schaffer and Kot, 1985). In the tradition of quantum theories, chaos theory has challenged the linear, mechanistic, cause and effect theories that have dominated scientific thinking. Chaos theory suggests that the Newtonian world view is too static, too reductionist, and is unable to explain the dynamic elements in all natural phenomena.The alternative put forward by quantum theorists was that in all phenomena there are linear and non-linear features, regularity and irregularity, order and chaos.

One example might help to illustrate the point more graphically. Chaos theory was applied by McQueen and Peskin (1983) to the workings of human heart valves. Earlier mechanistic models of heart function described the heart as a series of chambers with valves operating between them to control the flow of blood. This model, though accurate to a degree, paid little attention to the ways in which blood actually changed the surface of the heart in a dynamic and unpredictable way. Difficulties with the early designs of artificial heart valves arose with a failure to realise that they could not adjust to blood flow with the same degree of flexibility as human valves could.

It may be that quantum theories have not received the attention they deserve from disciplines such as speech and language therapy. For many years, clinicians have struggled to apply the 'linear' approach, perhaps without being aware that there was an alternative paradigm which had created a revolution in other fields of enquiry. Speech and language therapists have long accepted that not all behaviours follow a linear course. For example, take the case of the therapist who assesses a client and comes to a conclusion about his or her communication. A few months later, they meet in a different context, and the client's way of communicating is totally different. Was the therapist's first assessment incorrect? Probably not. But it was limited in that the assessment in the first context could not predict the client's behaviour in the second.

What quantum theory brings is an acceptance that there is a non-linearity in all natural phenomena. An acceptance of the principle of regularity and irregularity at work in all mechanisms – that some patterns are orderly in space but not orderly in time, and that there are static and oscillating, stable and unstable forces at work within the same mechanisms – can change the way in which one looks at the world.

Psychology

Psychology has also experienced radical paradigm shifts in its history. The early writings of William James (1890) who pursued a self-analytical, introspective approach in his attempts to unravel the mysteries of the human mind were followed by the behaviourists (Watson, 1919; Skinner, 1938), who suggested that human behaviour should be the sole subject matter of psychology. This shift was accompanied by a desire for measurement which is still very much with us. They were followed by the cognitive psychologists (e.g. Neisser, 1967) who considered behaviourism too simplistic. Neisser and others were interested in internal mental processes such as perception, memory, problem solving , imagery and memory. Still more recent developments are the humanistic and culturally driven theories of human behaviour, which emphasise the interaction between people and their present environments (Rogers, 1951; Egan, 1990).

These paradigm shifts have not followed a linear route, however. For example, at about the same time that the behaviourists were preoccupied with their experiments into extrinsic cause and effect relationships, Freud and his colleagues were asserting that human behaviour was driven not by outside stimuli but by innate instincts, unconscious processes, thoughts, fears and desires.

Linguistics

Similar trends can be observed in the history of linguistics. Up until the early 1930s, 'traditional grammar' was essentially descriptive and largely unsystematic. A new way of thinking about language was developed by the structuralists, led by Bloomfield (1933). This led to a more rigorous and principled treatment of the various phenomena of language. Language was seen as a series of subsystems, such as phonology, syntax and semantics, each obeying its own specific rules and principles. This culminated in the Chomskian revolution, which sought to explain as well as describe linguistic phenomena (Chomsky, 1965). Generative grammar saw syntax as the central, productive component of language, and language was studied in a decontextualised way.

Parallel to this but independently of it, researchers became interested in the social and functional aspects of language and for some time a tension existed between the so-called pure linguists and those interested in language use. The study of pragmatics was born. In the last few years, more linguists have seen the study of language as necessarily including pragmatics, acknowledging the fact that linguistic phenomena can only be explained with reference to pragmatic principles (see Chapter 8 for further discussion).

Speech and language therapy

The history of speech and language therapy follows a similarly winding pathway through its own shifting paradigms. The early speech correctionists were pioneers and experimenters who were concerned with either voice and speech projection, or with remediation of voice or speech. They were sometimes a little wild in their experimentation. In 1925, Travis conducted one of the first recorded experiments in 'speech correction'. He fired a blank pistol with no warning over the head of a stutterer, and compared the stutterer's speech against his recording of 'normal' speech production (presumably a normal speaker also had a pistol fired over his head under similar circumstances). This type of experimentation, which today seems quite outrageous, was at that time a serious attempt to understand more about the causes of speech difficulty. Since those early days, the profession has developed into something of a polymath profession, addressing the communication needs of many different groups of people and using many different methods to achieve this (hopefully without gunfire). Speech and language therapy is no longer concerned only with speech and voice problems – it engages in intervention for every type of communication difficulty, from acquired aphasia to developmental language delay.

As a result of its growing involvement in so many different types of communication difficulty, the speech and language therapy profession has been influenced by the paradigm shifts in the related disciplines of psychology and linguistics. One such shift has been away from behaviourism in the form of behaviour modification techniques (Ryan, 1971; Ryan and van Kirk, 1974) or measuring MLUs (mean length of utterances) to a more interpretative approach, focusing on the therapeutic relationship (Rogers, 1951; Egan, 1990), and on the nature of interactions (Austin, 1962; Hymes, 1971; Halliday, 1978; Gumperz, 1982).

It is no coincidence that speech and language therapy services, which have traditionally concentrated on intrinsic aspects of the client's communication, are now focusing on the extrinsic factors in the client's environment. Speech and language therapists are increasingly emphasising that communication skills cannot be taught in isolation from the client's everyday social context, and therefore the values and perceptions of carers are of great importance to bringing about changes. It could be argued that this shift from intrinsic to extrinsic influences runs in parallel with the shifts in clinical linguistics from syntactic to pragmatic approaches, and in psychology from behaviourism to psychodynamic approaches.

Learning disabilities

The history of change in the field of learning disabilities is no less colourful. It is beyond the scope of this book to specify in detail the changes that have taken place; however, the interested reader is referred to Ryan and Thomas, (1987) for an illuminating account of the subject.

The major paradigm shift in services for people with learning disabilities has been from a protectionist, containment approach, characterised by institutions for people with learning disabilities, to an approach driven by rights to self-determination and rights to an 'ordinary life' in ordinary community settings (White Paper, 1971; Kings Fund, 1980; Jay Report, 1979). This protectionism has its roots in society's negative perception of people with disabilities as 'abnormal', 'evil' or 'holy innocents' 'in need of protection and care'. Hence the need arose for institutions in which people with disabilities could live together, forever 'protected' from society (Morris, 1969; Townsend, 1969). This kind of segregation was commonplace in the UK until the 1970s, when the political climate began to change. This came about because people with disabilities were themselves finding a voice and protesting that they did not wish to continue living segregated lives (Kings Fund, 1984; CMH, 1986). The changes also came about because research into the negative consequences of institutional life was receiving more attention (Zigler, 1961; King, Raynes and Tizard, 1971; Zigler and Balla 1972; Oswin, 1978; Tyne, 1978). The horrors of life in large mental hospitals were coming to the attention of the media; for example, the Ely Inquiry (HMSO, 1969), and later reports by Shearer (1976), the Normansfield Hospital Report (1978), and the National Development Group Reports (1978, 1984) did much to alter public opinion and subsequently influence government policy (Martin, 1984). In addition, Wolfensberger and his colleagues were advocating that services to people with learning disabilities should be directed by the principle that individuals have rights – rights to ordinary life experiences, rights to additional help and support which allow such experiences to occur, and rights to be valued by the society as individuals not as 'the handicapped' (Nirje, 1969; Wolfensberger, 1972; O'Brien, 1981). These issues are discussed in more detail in Chapter 6. What is important in this context is that major changes were and still are taking place, in people's attitudes to individuals with learning disabilities (Table 1.1). At best, they are no longer a silent, segregated group, patronised by society's sometimes hostile, sometimes benevolent attitudes. They are individuals, interacting, demanding, learning and enjoying the same ordinary life experiences as other members of society. At worst, they are somewhere along the road towards living those experiences.

Table 1.1 Paradigm shifts in linguistics and psychology, speech and language therapy and services to people with learning disabilities

Psychology	Introspection	Behaviourism	Psychodynamic approaches
Linguistics	Descriptive	Structuralist and generative	Pragmatics
Speech therapy	Speech correction	Phonology/syntax semantics	Functional approaches
Services to people with learning disabilities	'Evil'	'Protect' the 'handicapped'	Living ordinary lives

Speech and Language Therapy and Learning Disabilities

McLaren and Bryson's (1987) review of recent epidemiological studies of learning disability concludes that the prevalence of severe and mild learning disability is generally 3–4 per 1000 of the population. However, prevalence figures for communication difficulty among the adult learning-disabled are not well documented. In 1982, Hallas, Fraser and MacGillivray suggested that the 'commonest and least treated disability' among people with learning disabilities was communication disorder. There are few studies which actually give prevalence figures to support this observation, however. McQueen et al. (1987) estimated that 66% of their learning-disabled population had some form of speech and language problem. Enderby and Davies (1989) estimated that as much as 50% of the population of learning-disabled adults in the UK would have some form of communication difficulty. However, surveys carried out in different parts of the UK suggest that between 73 and 89% of the population have an identified communication difficulty. For example, Budd's (1981) survey of the adult learning-disabled population in Nottinghamshire revealed that 73% had communication problems. Parker and Liddle (1987) found that 78% of the adult learning-disabled population in west Berkshire had communication difficulties. Noble's (1990) detailed study of the population of one day centre in Avon concluded that 89% had communication difficulties that 'required speech and language therapy'. Enderby and Davies' (1989) estimate of 50% may be quite conservative.

Enderby and Davies also estimated that almost a third of all speech and language therapy resources in the UK were directed at the learning-disabled population. The Manpower Planning Advisory Group Report (1990), in their review of speech and language therapy manpower in the UK, estimated that clients with learning disabilities represented the second largest group of people requiring speech and language therapy services. This constituted 17% of total speech and language therapy staffing levels. There will, however, be considerable variation in the amount of provision in different parts of the country. For example, Dobson (1990) in her survey of speech and language therapy services to adults with learning disabilities in 15 UK health districts, found that the level of staffing varied from 1 full-time equivalent per 100 000 to 0.15 full-time equivalent per 100 000.

There has undoubtedly been an increase in the number of therapists working with adults with learning disabilities over the last 10 years. Some would argue that this has had more to do with the increased demand for services than with the development of new precepts about what speech and language therapy actually has to offer this client group. To date, there is certainly very little published work on speech and language therapy's contribution to learning disabilities. There used to be very little specific teaching on learning disabilities at undergraduate and graduate level. Enderby, Simpson and Wheeler (1992), in their review of therapy services to adults with learning disabilities in the south-west of England, reported that therapists felt they were ill-prepared as undergraduates for the 'practical implementation of therapy for this client group'. Unfortunately, no comparisons with other client groups were available.

Enderby and Davies (1989) suggested that the boundaries around the speech and language therapy profession have expanded far beyond its capacity to supply adequate services, partly because the profession itself has little idea of when and how to impose these boundaries. However, this may not simply be a supply and demand issue. Many speech and language therapists argue, rightly or wrongly, that they have chosen to work in the learning disabilities field because the philosophy that underpins services to people with learning disabilities is one which they embrace more readily than the more medically or developmentally orientated philosophies of some of their speech and language therapy colleagues (medical philosophy in this context refers to a disease-orientated approach, and the developmental philosophy to the use of developmental norms as a basis for planning intervention). This philosophy, they argue, is a more reasoned starting point for speech and language therapy intervention, a more practical approach to working with people who are not 'ill', and are not 'children'.

Speech and language therapists working with people with learning disabilities have moved outside the medical and developmental frameworks and into a different theoretical framework. What are the consequences of this? Rejection of the medical and developmental frameworks has resulted in a polarisation of views on which theories are acceptable and which are unacceptable. For example, many clinicians now believe that linguistics has virtually nothing to contribute to our understanding of the communication of adults with learning disabilities, because all that matters is language in use, or pragmatics. This argument assumes that pragmatics and linguistics have little or nothing to do with each other. We would argue that this is a forced theoretical dichotomy that bears very little relation to either an authentic understanding of the subject or the realities of communication in context, an issue that will be addressed in more detail in later chapters.

Another polarisation of views which clouds the field is that medical and sociological approaches to working with adults with learning disabilities are somehow in opposition to each other. We would suggest that medical knowledge, for example, knowledge of the causes and cures for hearing impairment, are extremely relevant to the lives of adults with learning disabilities, not least because the incidence of hearing loss is so high (Nolan et al., 1980; Yeates, 1980). The application of medical knowledge is no less relevant to adults with learning disabilities than it is to any other member of society.

The speech and language therapy profession may not yet have found a resting place for itself within the theories and philosophies which have developed around learning disabilities. This book is an attempt to explore some of the theories, to examine the role and contribution of the speech therapist, to ask questions which are pertinent to the work of the speech therapist, and hopefully to generate further systematic enquiry into this specialist area of practice. The tenets which are central to this relatively new area include the principles of normalisation, the psychosocial approach to intervention and the multidimensional approach to assessment and intervention. The book also argues that the development of evaluative research using qualitative and quantitative methods is essential to the development of the discipline, and that in this field, as in any other, replication of research findings is the key to progress.

Book Outline

This chapter has given an introduction to some of the ideas that have influenced the writing of this book. The chapters which follow will hopefully give substance to these ideas. The book is divided into three parts. The first part examines current assessment issues, the second part concerns itself with management issues and the third with future directions in communication assessment and research. Chapters 2 and 3 discuss the principles of communication assessment in some detail, questioning the validity of using assessments designed for other groups with this client group. Chapter 4 gives a description of four communication assessment procedures that have been designed specifically for use with learning-disabled adults.

In the second part of the book the reader is asked to consider management issues, first from the viewpoint of the client, exploring some of the common experiences of people with learning disabilities and how these might have an influence on the use of communication, and secondly from the viewpoint of the therapist. There follows a focus on the features of the communication environment that can influence communication. A discussion of the People in Systems theory and how it might be related to the study of the communication environment is provided.

The following two chapters examine issues in service delivery. The centrality of the principle of normalisation, the influence of the self-advocacy movement and the changing patterns of health and social care delivery are outlined. Examples are given of the different environments in which practitioners might find themselves. Models of good practice in different areas of intervention are discussed. More specific guidelines on how to decide which clients should be seen and on what basis, how to measure changes over time in a client's progress, and how to work with speech and language therapy assistants are also given here. The importance of staff training, systematically and sensitively delivered, is also discussed.

In the final part of the book, future directions in communication assessment and research are discussed. Chapter 8 presents an alternative way of examining communication using an integrated pragmatic and linguistic framework. Chapter 9 raises questions about accountability, gives examples of research methods and outcomes relevant to adults. Both these chapters emphasise the need for more research into the communicative abilities of adults with learning disabilities.

Chapter 2
Issues in Assessment

Language or, increasingly, communication assessments are carried out in a variety of fields and for a variety of purposes. The purposes can range from the purely theoretical to the purely practical. For example, psycholinguistic tests, whose purpose is to identify the nature of linguistic representations and linguistic or communicative processes, cluster at the purely theoretical end of the range, whereas assessments carried out with the aim of diagnosing language impairment clearly fall towards the practical end. The aims and methods may be different but they do not represent an irreconcilable dichotomy. The results of psycholinguistic testing must inform the design of practical assessments and vice versa. Even within the more practically orientated assessments we find a wide range of purposes. Communication assessments are used in schools, both in native-language and foreign-language teaching, (Davies, 1990; *Language Testing*, 1984). The purpose here may be selecting, streaming, grading or for evaluating progress, for comparing the relative efficiency of different teaching methods, or for the most obvious pedagogical purpose of determining 'what to teach next'. Language assessments are also used widely with normal adult populations. Their results can have important implications in the context of job applications and promotion (e.g. The Language Usage subtest of The General Clerical Test, 1992). This may be completely informal or contain specific tests, especially where people from different ethnic backgrounds are involved. And finally, and for the present text perhaps most importantly, communication assessments are carried out in speech and language therapy, both in adult and child populations, in order to to screen, diagnose, evaluate progress and to design intervention programmes, if communication is deemed less than adequate.

Why should speech and language therapists assess the communication of adults with learning disabilities? At first reading, the inevitable answer to this question may look like an attempt to state the obvious, but given that attitudes towards adults with learning disabilities run along a continuum from 'There is nothing more that can be done for these people – they cannot learn anything new' to 'Adults with learning disabilities are just the same as the rest of us!', it is worth considering for a moment just why speech and language therapists are involved with this population at all.

First, speech and language therapists are communication specialists and, as such, provide a service to any member of society with a communication difficulty. The role of the speech and language therapist is to assess and diagnose the communication difficulty, and to provide therapy where appropriate. People with learning difficulties have the same right of access to that service as other people with communication difficulties (Wolfensberger, 1972; O'Brien and Tyne, 1981).

Secondly, as discussed in the previous chapter, there is both an identified need and a demand for speech and language therapy expertise (Budd, 1981; Parker and Liddle, 1987; Noble 1990). On the demand side, there is evidence that staff who work with adults with learning disabilities do recognise that speech and language therapy is a valuable service. For example, in a survey of adult training centres in England and Wales, staff placed speech and language therapists as the highest priority on their list of professional help required (Whelan and Speake 1977). Perhaps more revealing still is this example from the Lanarkshire Social Services Report on Day Services to People with Learning Difficulties (1985). The Working Party was made up of parents and professionals, and was brought together by Lanarkshire Social Services Department in an attempt to identify the needs of people with learning disabilities in concrete and practical ways. Among other issues addressed, the Working Party asked: 'What do people with learning difficulties need to learn in order to live independently in the community?' Three core requirements were identified:

1. An understanding of social conventions and appropriate behaviours.
2. A general preparation for independent living.
3. An emphasis on increasing communication skills and insights into the nature of social relationships.

The references to communication skills being central to the development of the skills necessary to living independently is the issue of relevance here. It is widely recognised that communication skills are the key that can unlock the door to living a more independent life. Other service providers recognise this only too well. Service users are beginning to express it for themselves and for their friends who cannot communicate.

Research into service users' perceptions of speech and language therapy services confirms this view. Recently, van der Gaag and Davies (1992c) used postal questionnaires to obtain the view of speech and language therapy service users in six health districts in the UK. They were asked to rate the speech and language therapy services in their respective day centres or schools. The learning-disabled users and their families were unanimous in their request for more speech and language therapy input.

What Are We Assessing?

The very existence of communication assessments relies on two tacit assumptions. One is that there is such a thing as optimal communicative proficiency, and the second, which is implied by this, is that communicative proficiency is measurable or even scorable.

Communicative proficiency

The notion of communicative proficiency is widely used in the literature on foreign language learning. It is similar to the concept of communicative competence as introduced by Hymes (1972), but it involves, additionally, some degree of value judgement as regards an individual's ability to mobilise his or her linguistic, sociolinguistic and discourse competence effectively (Ingram, 1985). A proficient communicator is, in other words, an effective communicator. The term communicative proficiency is not explicitly adopted in speech and language therapy, although evaluation of communicative abilities implies this concept implicitly. We shall adopt the somewhat less loaded terms 'communicative efficiency' or 'communicative effectiveness' for more or less the same concept. As we shall be pointing out, this involves both linguistic and non-linguistic skills. Often an additional competence is added to these, namely 'strategic' competence, which is defined as the ability to use strategies for making the best use of what one knows about how a language works, in order to interpret, express and negotiate meaning in a given context (Savignon, 1985).

Communication

As a first step in examining the notion of communicative effectiveness a distinction will be made between communication, language and linguistic communication. 'Language and communication are often seen as two sides of the same coin. On this view the essential feature of language is that it is used for communication, and the essential feature of communication is that it involves the use of language or a code' (Sperber and Wilson, 1986, p. 173). In fact we know that this is not the case. Language is not indispensable for communication and, conversely, languages exist for purposes other than communication.

What is communication? Communication is conveying some message a communicator has in mind, and its interpretation by an addressee. The message can be assumptions, beliefs, wishes, feelings etc. Its purpose can be information sharing, eliciting information, promising, threatening, warning or social. We shall be expanding on these in a later part of the chapter. What communication necessarily involves is the expression, interpretation and negotiation of meaning, involving interaction between two or more persons in context. A raised eyebrow can indicate a request for repetition, questioning, surprise, doubt or disbelief in one type of context, or greeting in another. It could even be a prearranged warning signal in yet another. Or it could just be a nervous tic. The different meanings listed above are not mutually exclusive and more than one of them can be conveyed at the same time. On the other hand, none of the above meanings is guaranteed by the raised eyebrow, save for the prearranged signal. In this sense non-linguistic communication can be said to be weak communication. In language each linguistic unit has at least a defined default value which is likely to be interpreted by all speakers as the same. However, the various manifestations of non-verbal communication are much more flexible. Consequently, they function much more as signs rather than codes. It is in the nature of non-coded stimuli that they 'tend to form a continuous range of variants' (Sperber and Wilson, 1986, p.175). Their interpretation is dependent on the addressee's ability to make inferences on the basis of his or her knowledge of the communicator and his or her knowledge of the world.

Non-linguistic communication is weak communication for a second reason, too. The range of potential meanings that can be expressed is very limited. They are constrained within the here and now. The meanings communicated can only be those which can either be enacted or pointed to. The following communication between a mother and her child could not be expressed, for example, by gestures: 'If you had listened to me you wouldn't have hurt yourself'.

It is not our intention to belittle the power of non-linguistic communication, but it is important to acknowledge that it has limitations, and it is desirable to establish what these limitations are.

Language

What is language? Introductory textbooks on linguistics all agree that the essential defining feature of language is that it is a set of codes to mentally represent meaning. This is not the same as to communicate meaning. Halliday (1970) distinguishes between three different functions of language, and terms these ideational, interpersonal and textual. Of these only the interpersonal and, arguably, the textual function have a communicative dimension. In discussing the ideational function he states: 'we use language to represent our experience of the processes, persons, objects, abstractions, qualities, states and relations of the world around us and inside us. ....hence 'ideational function' (Halliday,

1970). A number of alternative terms have been used for this same function, namely representational, cognitive, semantic, factual–notional and experiential.

A similar view is expressed by Sperber and Wilson: language is a set of semantically interpreted well-formed formulas. It is an essential tool for the processing and memorising of information. 'The activities which necessarily involve the use of language are not communicative but cognitive' (Sperber and Wilson, 1986, p.173.) They go on to say that the fact that language and communication can be found together in humans, that humans have developed languages which can be used for communication 'tells us nothing about the essential nature of language' (p.173). But most importantly, they note: 'The originality of the human species is precisely to have found this curious additional use for something which many other species also possess' (p.173) rather like 'the originality of elephants is that they can use their noses for the curious additional purpose of picking things up....However, it is as strange for humans to conclude that the essential purpose of language is for communication as it would be for elephants to conclude that the essential purpose of noses is for picking things up' (p. 173). But, of course, just as the elephant's nose has been adapted for its additional function, so human language differs from other forms of communication in that it has also been adapted to its communicative function. Over the course of evolution language and communication have often become inseparable. In order to establish how they interact, however, it is necessary to understand the difference between the two.

Linguistic communication

In the course of non-linguistic communication almost any sign can be communicative, provided the addressee can make the appropriate inferences. The earlier example of the raised eyebrow is just one illustration. The inferences concern the communicator's possible motivation for making a sign, and the interpretation of this in the given context. In linguistic communication the meaning of an utterance, though not necessarily the message to be conveyed, is determined by the codes or formulas it contains. There is no continuity or simultaneous representation of several meanings. Even in the case of ambiguous sentences, as, for example, in 'The police cannot stop drinking in Scotland', a choice of several alternative meanings is made. There is no overlap. This does not mean, however, that linguistic codes are perfectly precise representations of thoughts, feelings, qualities etc. There are expressions that are vague. For example the terms 'doctor', 'patient', 'therapist', or 'client' are vague as to gender , whereas in other cases gender is explicitly expressed, e.g. compare 'actor' with 'actress'. Many terms that denote qualities are not possible to interpret out of context.

Take the term 'large', it is not possible to understand exactly what size is meant by this word if one does not know what entity it applies to. A large elephant is likely to be considerably larger than a large mouse, but considerably smaller than a small hill. In addition, when language is used in communication, the literal meaning of an utterance does not necessarily correspond to the message it can convey. For example, if someone says: 'I'm boiling', he most certainly does not mean 'boiling' literally, otherwise he would not be in a position to say it. He might be conveying one of a number of possible messages, such as: 'turn the heating down', 'could someone open the window?', 'why are we wasting gas?', 'I do not feel like working' and others.

In order to perceive the message that a communicative utterance conveys, listeners must first of all possess the linguistic codes to decode the utterance. Although a great variety of different messages can be conveyed by a particular sentence these are not infinite, and not totally random. The linguistic form, together with cultural and social conventions, constrains the range of possible messages. For example, none of the above messages would have been yielded by uttering the sentence: 'It is freezing cold here'. In addition to decoding the utterances, listeners also need to make inferences, in a similar way as in non-linguistic communication. The difference is that their choices are more strictly guided by the linguistic codes. 'The linguistic description of an utterance is determined by grammar. This linguistic description yields a range of semantic representations. Each semantic representation is a schema which must be completed and integrated into an assumption about the speaker's informative intention' (Sperber and Wilson, 1986, p. 175). This is true whether language is transmitted by the oral/auditory channel, through the medium of writing or by sign language.

A qualitative comparison of non-linguistic and linguistic communication inevitably leads to the conclusion that when language and other forms of communication come together the outcome is a superior form of communication. Despite the fact that the linguistic analysis of an utterance underdetermines its interpretation, a remarkable degree of precision and complexity can be achieved which is not paralleled in any other form of communication that does not involve language.

In addition to the greater precision, the range of meanings is greatly increased. This is partly due to the fact that the linguistic code is abstracted away from the physical world and is capable of encoding totally abstract meanings. It enables communication which is divorced from the here and now, and it is capable of representing hypothetical situations. By combining basic vocabulary items into complex structures it is capable of representing much more complex concepts and relationships than its non-linguistic counterpart. Many of the features which are used in non-linguistic communication can be utilised in linguistic communication. Such paralinguistic features as intonation, volume and duration can be superimposed on the linguistic form to add further to the range of meanings that can be conveyed. It can be said that verbal communication is a specifically human enhancement of any non-coded communication. Nobody who has ever tried to exist in a language environment other than his or her own can fail to appreciate the immense power of non-verbal communication at the same time as lament its miserable limitations.

Evidence for the distinction between language and communication.

These distinctions between communication and language, made on theoretical grounds, are well supported by empirical facts. Perhaps the most frequently observed is the double dissociation between linguistic and non-linguistic communicative abilities. The language of spina bifida children with so called 'cocktail party syndrome' is a good example of language which is clearly articulated, makes use of wide range of complex syntactic structures and a sizeable vocabulary, but which fails to communicate (Tew, 1979). Young children with normal language development spend a great deal of their time talking to themselves, and even stop doing so when someone enters the room (Weir, 1962; Vygotsky, 1986). Their use of language can hardly be regarded as communicative.

On the other side of the coin, it has been shown that low Token Test scores and well preserved communicative abilities in aphasic patients can and often do co-occur. At the same time, high Token Test scores are not predictive of high-level communicative abilities. Rondall and Lambert (1983) also observed this dissociation in their analysis of conversations between a group of moderately and severely mentally handicapped adults and familiar non-handicapped adults. They found that the adults were able to convey meanings despite the 'severe formal restrictions in their use of syntactic structures'. Sollenberger (1978), in a discussion on foreign language learning, shows how this dissociation can happen the other way as well. A person's language proficiency, although it may be accurate enough in purely linguistic terms, does not guarantee effective communication: 'In some cases, it may enable a person to misinterpret or foul up more effectively... I'm sure we all know people who talk nonsense fluently. On the other hand, I know people who butcher language, whose accents are atrocious and whose vocabularies are limited. For these reasons we give them low proficiency ratings. Yet, for some reason, some of them are effective communicators.'

Components of Effective Communication

Bearing these distinctions in mind, and accepting the superiority of verbal communication, how can we characterise the factors that influence communication and how can we measure communicative effectiveness?

Earlier, communication was defined very broadly as the conveying of some meaning a communicator or speaker has in mind, and its interpretation by an addressee or listener, in context. In fact, the context includes the communicator and the addressee (for the sake of ease of expression we shall be using the terms 'speaker' and 'listener', irrespective of whether we talk about linguistic communication through the oral, written or sign medium, or non-linguistic communication). Accordingly, the following components of communication will be discussed in some detail: meanings conveyed: topics and functions of communication; context: participants, the communicative situation and the medium of communication. It is important to note that all components interact with each other in the course of communication, continuously selecting and shaping both the amount and style of language used.

Meanings conveyed

Types of meaning, in this context, can be considered from two different points of view. These are the types of topics a speaker wishes to communicate about, and the set of communicative functions.

Topic of communication

It is virtually impossible to provide an exhaustive list of all imaginable topics speakers may want to communicate about. However, as a first step in trying to identify at least some, it would appear sensible to look into the vocabulary. Words are the most obvious codes for the types of meaning language encodes. It is one of the ongoing concerns of semantics to attempt to classify topics to reflect the way the vocabulary is organised. One way in which this is done in contemporary linguistics is to regard the meaning of words as classifiable in terms of semantic fields (Lyons, 1977; Crystal, 1982). Different linguists slice up the cake differently. None of the attempts so far has satisfied all. For one thing, they inevitably fall short of being complete. In addition, the division of topics into major semantic classes and subclasses often appears somewhat arbitrary, though undoubtedly of use for analytical purposes. Crystal (1982), for example, lists 12 major themes: human form and function, activity, sensory, leisure, transport, fauna, flora and elements, domestic setting, dimensions, institutions and the world. These are further subdivided into 61 major semantic fields, each with additional subclasses.

Topics are closely bound up with the type of situation in which communication takes place. On the one hand, the assignment of a word to a particular semantic field is determined by the context. The word 'car' would normally be assigned to transport, but when talking about the outcome of an accident where a pedestrian was hit by a car, it might be better to assign it to human form and function. It is, of course, not necessary to adhere rigidly to any one author's classification of themes. Therapists and carers, no doubt, are capable of identifying the topic of any one communicative event. On the other hand, the situation might determine the topic. For example, when buying a season ticket for British Rail, only a very restricted range of topics are appropriate. Anything that deviated from the 'business in hand' would be regarded as odd by the railway clerk, and a positive nuisance by the long queue of people also trying to buy a season ticket. At a party, on the other hand, virtually anything goes, including the topic of buying a season ticket. The notion of communicative situation will be discussed in some detail in the section entitled 'Context'.

Another approach to classifying meanings is in terms of the kinds of concepts and conceptual structures that utterances reflect, (Jackendoff, 1983).The details of these will be taken up in Chapter 8, but it is possible to give a brief summary here. Essentially, utterances are about events, states, properties and entities that participate in the events and states, or whose properties the utterance relates to. Additional basic concepts encoded in language are location (both spatial and temporal, static and dynamic), possession, identification and quantity.

It is important to note that the two approaches are not mutually exclusive. Rather, the conceptual structure approach subsumes the semantic field approach, in that it deals with meaning on a more general level. Furthermore, it provides a direct link between cognitive processes and their reflection in the organisation of language, irrespective of world knowledge or experience. Therefore, it may well be a more appropriate model to start with in order to capture abilities relating to verbal communication per se, rather than those abilities that are dependent on highly idiosyncratic personal experience.

Communicative functions

This term refers to the various purposes that give rise to communicative acts. They have been studied widely in anthropology, philosophy, sociolinguistics and pragmatics. The term comes in various guises, for example communicative functions (Leech and Svartvik, 1975), communicative intentions (Sperber and Wilson, 1986), or illocutionary acts (Austin, 1962; Searle, 1969) to mention just a few.

As in all classifications, so too in the classification of communicative functions a decision has to be made as to the degree of detail. A carefully balanced compromise must be found between completeness on the one hand and unwieldiness on the other. We cannot hope to give an exhaustive list of the functions, but we can indicate the range they cover.

Broadly speaking, it is possible to classify communicative functions into two major types. These are (Brown and Yule, 1983): the *transactional* and the *interactional* functions. Although this division is a useful one, particularly for analytical purposes, the dividing line is not a sharp one. Often communicative acts contain elements of both in varying proportions, but one almost always predominates over the other.

The transactional function of language primarily serves the transference of 'factual' information. It is essentially propositional in nature, i.e. the speaker formulates propositions which the listener retrieves from the utterance. Factual information can be about actual facts, or at least facts as the speaker believes them to be true. Typical examples are giving instructions as to how to get from A to B, describing a traffic accident, giving a report about some event or person, telling a doctor about one's symptoms, description of goods and services or delivering a lecture, say, on the functions of language. It can also be about physical, psychological or mental states such as headaches, tiredness, fitness, comfort and discomfort, or happiness, sadness, desires, love, hate, worry, or certainty, uncertainty, imaginings, beliefs etc. Information can also relate to attitudes to facts or assumed facts, for example, interest, pleasure, surprise, doubt, disbelief, preference, hope, regret, approval, disapproval, concern, sympathy. In addition to facts attitudes can also relate to text, i.e. what the previous speaker has just said.

The transactional functions of language can take the form of giving or requesting information. Giving information can be spontaneous (self-initiated) or elicited. In either case there is an assumption on the speaker's part that listeners do not have the information and that it is in their or the speaker's interest that they should have it. In requesting information the speaker inevitably also informs listeners that there is something they do not know, and that they ascribe this knowledge to the speaker. This may be an important factor to remember when assessing the communication skills of adults with learning disabilities. People with low self-esteem are often reticent when it comes to asking questions: it can look like an admission of inferiority, or an admission of dependence.

A third form of communication is wedged in between the transactional and interactional functions, and this is to influence the behaviour of other people. This can be manifested in commands to carry out instructions, requests for services, advice to act in a certain manner, warning, promising or threatening.

The primarily interactional function of language serves social relationships rather than the transference of information. It can serve the establishment, maintenance or severance of such relationships. Typical examples are greetings, farewells, thanks, apologies, good wishes, congratulations and the kind of conversations that surround purchases in one's local shops, in the pub, or whenever people happen to find themselves in some shared situation with time on their hands, such as waiting rooms, bus stops, train journeys and the like. It is this function of language that serves to establish role relationships and social belonging. Sociologists and anthropologists attach enormous importance to this function. Brown and Yule summarise it as follows 'It is clearly the case that a great deal of everyday human interaction is characterised by the primarily interpersonal rather than the primarily transactional use of language' (Brown and Yule, 1983, p. 3).

Context

The notion of context is treated differently by different authors in the literature. It can have an all-inclusive interpretation, which involves absolutely everything in which the communicative act is embedded. Under this kind of interpretation the participants also form part of the context (e.g. Sperber and Wilson, 1986; Lyons, 1977; Ochs, 1979). We follow Ochs (1979): 'The scope of context is not easy to define... One must consider the social and psychological world in which the language user operates at any given time' (p.1); 'it includes minimally, language users' beliefs and assumptions about temporal, spatial, and social settings; prior, ongoing and future actions (verbal, non-verbal) and the state of knowledge and attentiveness of those participating in the social interaction in hand' (p.5).

Participants

The main protagonists in the communicative act are, of course, the participants. It is important to stress that communication is a two-way process involving at least a speaker and a listener. When people talk to their pet fish or their plants they are not, in fact, engaged in communicative behaviour. Speakers must be able to assess the personal relationship that holds between themselves and their listeners. This means knowing enough about the identity, background, status, interests and inclinations of the listener and also knowing enough about his or her shared knowledge of the world (Sperber and Wilson, 1986). The perceived role a speaker or a listener has in a communicative situation influences both the communicative functions and the manner in which communication takes place. For example, it would be totally inappropriate for a customer in a garage to give a lecture on the principles of the combustion engine to the car mechanic, as either he knows it, or at least he would like the pretence to be maintained that he knows it, but in any case the customer is the last person from whom he would ever wish to hear about it.

How much do speaker and listener need to know about each other? This is determined entirely by the communicative situation. Clearly one need not possess a great deal of personal knowledge about a shop-keeper in order to carry out a successful shopping transaction, but even in the shopping context the speaker/listener relationship can influence the kind of communication that takes place. For example, if a person always goes to the same newsagent and always buys the same paper, the content of the verbal communication can be restricted to merely exchanging greetings and the transaction itself: the handing over of the paper and the money may be accompanied by no speech at all. The opposite is illustrated by the following popular story about Sir Thomas Beecham, the well known conductor. Strolling along Piccadilly one day he was greeted by a very well dressed lady who congratulated him on the excellent performance the previous night, which both she and her brother enjoyed greatly. Sir Thomas, having thanked her for the compliment, proceeded to ask her: 'And what is your brother doing nowadays?' The reply to this was: 'Oh, he is still the King'.

The speaker clearly needs to know enough about the listener in order to choose the right topic, the right speech style, the right amount of language and the appropriate function. Whatever the context, the listener also needs to know enough about the speaker in order to make the necessary inferences as to the purpose of the communication and to interpret the message that was meant to be conveyed. The concept of familiarity is of special significance in the case of people with communication problems, as a greater degree of empathy might be needed on the part of the listener to make the right inferences.

In addition to the speaker/listener relationship and mutual knowledge, there are personality factors such as introversion, extroversion, temporary tiredness, mental states such as euphoria or depression, which all have a bearing on and influence communication.

Communicative situation

The temporal, spatial and social setting can also be termed the communicative situation. The range of situations in which various communicative functions are put to use varies greatly according to the circumstances in which people live. It is possible, however, to list some which are relevant to practically everybody who is able to lead an independent existence, say, in modern-day Britain. These include family situations, using various public facilities, finding one's way, the use of public transport, shopping transactions of all kinds, eating out, visits to the doctor or dentist, social gatherings, work place or school or day centres, use of the telephone or watching television.

The content and form of communication on the part of the speaker, as well as the interpretation of the intended message by the listener, are greatly determined by aspects of the communicative situation as they are perceived by the participants. Failure to assess correctly any one aspect of the context can lead to misunderstandings, which are not always as amusing as in the story told about a British diplomat, who went to an evening engagement in Vienna and found himself standing next to a voluptuous figure in a purple dress. He asked his neighbour: 'Shall we waltz?', to which the figure replied: 'There are three reasons why we should not waltz. One: this is a banquet and not a ball; two: the music is not a waltz but the Austrian national anthem; and three: I am the Archbishop of Salzburg'.

Medium of communication

Another important influencing contextual factor is the medium of communication. In the absence of language, various signs – bodily and facial gestures as well as non-linguistic sound – carry the burden of communication. It is quite often the case that the use of these is perfected to a considerable degree to compensate for lack of language. The limitations have already been mentioned and will be taken up again later.

If communication takes place through the medium of spoken language, then of course adequate knowledge of the language is a prerequisite of communicative efficiency. The linguistic skills include articulatory skills, fluency, vocabulary, syntactic structures and the ability to map semantic representations onto syntactic structures. A detailed outline of the linguistic skills and their communicative use will be given in Chapter 8. However, adequate knowledge of the language does not necessarily mean perfect knowledge of all of its component subsystems. One important property of language is its highly redundant nature. The knowledge of a particular discrete element is not indispensable in language use: the syntactic, discourse or semantic context may help the speaker or the listener to get by without it. The redundant nature of language is complemented by the psycholinguistic processing strategies listeners are able to employ. That is, on the basis of their knowledge of grammar they are able to set up 'expectancy grammars' for utterances they hear. This means calculated guesses at those parts of an utterance they missed for some reason or another. For example, imagine a hostess serving strawberries after dinner saying: 'I am frightfully sorry but the cat has eaten ...' at which point the noise of a supersonic aircraft blocks out her voice. The guests will be able to supply the missing word without a great deal of effort. The degree of redundancy in language is considerably increased when utterances are embedded in communicative contexts.

Evidence from psycholinguistic research has shown that listeners can identify words very rapidly even before a whole word has been uttered, and that such 'fast word recognitions' are strongly facilitated by the context in which the word appears. (Tyler and Wessels, 1983). In normal face-to-face interaction language is normally accompanied by extralinguistic signs, such as gestures. The use of these can further reduce the dependency on language.

The various components that make up communication have been listed and discussed. They all play a part and they are all interdependent. The secret of successful communication lies in a careful balancing and counterbalancing act involving the consideration of all the components listed and the ability to play off one component against another, should the need arise.

How Can We Measure Communicative Effectiveness?

It is one thing to identify what contributes to the effectiveness of communication but it is another thing to answer the question: what does it mean to communicate successfully? One perfectly sensible answer could be the following: if to communicate is to convey a message that a speaker has in mind, then the measure of success is the degree to which the message has been conveyed. But there is a problem here: how can we ever reliably know what the speaker had in mind? How can we tell if what we understood was indeed the intended message, or if it was all that was intended? The simple answer is that we can never know. In this sense there can be no realistic measure of communicative effectiveness. There is no absolute against which we can measure particular communicative events.

Sperber and Wilson (1986) provide a measure for communicative success, at least as far as individual utterances are concerned. An utterance is communicative to the extent that it enlarges the shared knowledge of the speaker and the listener. In other words, if the speaker is in possession of some information that the listener does not have, then passing on this information is of communicative value. So, for example the utterance 'It is raining' would be straightforwardly communicative in a situation where the addressee was about to take a party of children out for a picnic, provided he did not know that it was raining. The same utterance can be indirectly communicative if both speaker and listener knew that it was raining, for example as an answer to the question 'Shall we walk or take a bus?' In which case the message would be something like 'Let's take the bus' rather than the literal meaning of the utterance. And yet in a third context the very same utterance may have a merely interactional function, being an idle remark, simply to establish conversational rapport. Whatever 'message' is intended, it will only be successfully conveyed if both speaker and listener have the same perception of the context and each other's intentions, and are capable of making the appropriate inferences.

The factors that contribute to this potential perfect harmony in understanding are so complex that they are probably beyond experimental control. 'In fact, it is unlikely that a valid and reliable test of 'communicative competence' in the looser sense of ability to communicate is ever likely to be devised, and in that many things beyond language itself are entailed, it is probably not appropriate for the language tester to measure it' (Ingram, 1985, p.226). Communicative events, of course, generally consist of more than single utterances or single exchanges of utterance pairs. Again, for analytical purposes, some communicative events can be usefully evaluated by an utterance-by-utterance analysis. Indeed, this is the approach we shall be advocating in Chapter 8, always bearing in mind that, because of the redundancy in language and because of the concerted and overlapping way in which the different components of communication interact, it is unlikely that careful measurement of each component will yield a realistic score. The whole is much more than the sum of its parts.

Communicative needs

In normal everyday life, of course, we do not need to measure people's communicative abilities. We may form opinions based on intuition and on our tastes. We may say that X is a better communicator than Y, or we may say that X is a better communicator in one situation than in another, but we rarely seek to modify people's communicative abilities. This is clearly not the case in the speech and language therapist's dealings with clients who have communication difficulties. It is precisely the therapist's job to modify, improve or enhance the client's communicative abilities when they are deemed to be inadequate. But what constitutes inadequate communication? A client's communicative abilities can only be deemed inadequate if they do not meet his or her needs. The problem lies in knowing what these needs are. The moral dilemma is that, as the client is unable to tell us what his or her needs are, we have to decide them. The danger is that we may underestimate or overestimate these needs. In the first case we are patronising; in the second we might appear overbearing. The second case was nicely exemplified by an elderly stroke patient who was diagnosed as a global aphasic. A young and eager speech and language therapist was introduced to her by her doctor. When the doctor departed the patient put her hand on the therapist's arm and said: 'Don't worry about me dear, I can speak, I just don't want to. I'll speak alright when they let me go home'.

How can we establish what communicative needs are? It seems that there is a continuum of needs from the basic and minimal to what can be regarded as optimal. Even without establishing a ceiling measure for this 'optimal level' we know intuitively when communication is near it. We might be clearer on what the minimum needs are: these are the minimal needs of every individual for physical survival in a society. It is the therapist's or carer's task to determine what any one particular client's needs are, and what the realistic aims might be given the client's potential. It is not an easy task and carries an enormous amount of responsibility. It can only be approached by knowing the client, the client's circumstances and by appreciating the factors that contribute to communicative effectiveness.

It also means appreciating the fact that needs and wishes are not necessarily the same thing. If communication has to do with information sharing then, paradoxically, the better we know somebody the less we need to communicate. At least, the less we need to communicate on the very basic level. The example of the lack of need to communicate in the newsagent's shop illustrates this. At the same time, the more we know somebody the more we may wish to communicate, on levels that are beyond mere survival. This is where the distinction as well as the overlap between the transactional and interactional functions of language is of particular relevance.

The claim was made earlier that linguistic communication is superior to non-linguistic communication. Indeed, it is difficult to imagine how some of the communicative functions – transactional or interactional – can be fulfilled without the use of language. Certain elementary transactional communication can be achieved by gestures – pointing and the like. Similarly, certain gross interactive social communication can take place by body language. Affection, dislike, anger, fear can be mimicked, but communicating about such attitudes as hope, preference, regret, approval, concern, or about psychological and mental states is virtually impossible without language. The expression of subtle degrees of closeness or distance, the negotiating of role relationships, peer solidarity and the like cannot easily be achieved with gestures.

There is another, very important function that language serves. It was not listed among the communicative functions because it is seen as an inadvertent corollary to language behaviour. This is self-expression. The fact that people identify strongly with their language is something that is well documented in the sociolinguistic literature on language and power (for example, Inglehart and Woodward, 1972). Throughout history, occupying powers have regarded the imposition of their own language at the expense of the indigenous language of the occupied nation as top priority. Conversely, occupied nations and ethnic minorities have always been ready to protect, sometimes ferociously, their indigenous languages. Identification with language has an important psychological role within individuals, too. When we communicate we give away a great deal about ourselves. We open up our personalities in very subtle ways. Although some of this can be conveyed by our general behaviour, 'it is through language that our humanity is expressed' (Fromkin and Rodman, 1978). It is our belief that this function of language is equal to or, at worst, a close second to our survival needs.

Chapter 3
Communication
Assessment

If we do not have vision, we will not start. If we do not have realism, we will not finish.

Robin Green

What Do We Expect from Assessments?

We are now in the seemingly impossible position of knowing what makes up communication, knowing that some people are in need of help to develop their potential to communicate, and at the same time knowing that we cannot determine precisely their needs nor measure precisely their effectiveness. The question is: is this precision really necessary? Possibly not. Judgements on communicative effectiveness are naturally somewhat subjective, but this does not mean that they are unreliable. A number of studies have shown that inter-rater reliability can be quite impressive in subjective measures of verbal behaviour (for example, van der Gaag, 1988). In the context of second language testing Ingram goes as far as to state: 'subjectivity is necessitated by the sheer complexity and redundancy of language and its development and, though subjective, the approach is not impressionistic since it requires the deliberate matching of observing behaviour with the global descriptions of language behaviour' (Ingram, 1985, p.222). We would argue that as long as judgements are informed judgements, subjectivity is perfectly acceptable.

Subjective or objective, it remains true that some measure of communicative ability is necessary in order to design communication programmes, evaluate them and make decisions as to whether a client needs therapy. In order to evaluate the available assessment procedures, we need to establish the criteria they must meet.

Tests or Assessments?

At first it might be helpful to try and dispel an unhelpful dichotomy between tests and assessments. 'Language testing is based on educational testing which itself derives from measurement theory and practice in psychology and psychometrics' (Davies, 1990 p.10). In psychology, testing is seen as an instrument of research. It is used to measure all kinds of behaviour. Tests can either have a theoretical or an applied focus. The theoretical aim of testing is to arrive at generalisations from the behaviour of individuals. This in turn leads to theories where the test results constitute the empirical evidence to support the theory. The practical aim of testing is to identify individual behaviour patterns with reference to some existing theory.

There are a number of problems with the term 'test'. One is that it is ambiguous. In fact it is used for two different purposes in assessment: one relates to the tasks which are designed to yield data, and the other to the process of evaluation. As far as the first of these is concerned, a test fulfils its purpose if it yields a sample of behaviour from which realistic predictions and generalisations can be made as to a person's general underlying abilities (Ingram, 1985; Savignon, 1985). The reason why tests, in this sense, are designed at all is purely practical. One such practical reason is that most behaviours, and communicative behaviours in particular, are enormously complex. In order to investigate the quality of communicative behaviour, be it for research purposes or with therapeutic aims in mind, it is often necessary to focus on one part of it while holding all the others constant. This is the only way in which the contribution of one part in relation to the whole can be measured, and to achieve this, tasks have to be designed artificially.

Another practical reason has to do with the time available to make judgements. The natural occurrence of any one communicative activity is dependent on factors which are outside the investigator's control. As the purpose of tests is to yield representative samples of behaviour from which generalisations can be made, it is necessary to elicit certain behaviours through set tasks.

The other aspect of testing concerns evaluation. It does not necessarily depend on 'test'-like tasks or data elicited in a 'test'-like situation. In practice, however, the two are often linked, for example, in standardised assessments. In this sense, all standardised assessments are tests. The assessments which are not based on test like-tasks, i.e. the ones that evaluate either totally naturally occurring behaviours or elicited naturalistic conversations have their own problems too, as will be discussed later. It could be argued that testing is involved even in these instances if we accept that, in its broadest sense, testing simply means evaluation. The only real difference between evaluations based on naturally occurring behaviours and the types of tests most other assessment procedures employ concerns the content and, specifically, the amount of interference or control in eliciting the behaviour. In the overview of methods currently used to assess communicative abilities in adults with learning disabilities, the term 'test' will be used when referring to assessment procedures that involve controlled elicitation of behaviour through tasks. Otherwise the more neutral term 'assessment procedure' will be adopted.

Core requirements of communication assessment procedures

It is now possible to discuss the core requirements of assessment procedures with particular reference to their applicability in assessing communication in adults with learning disabilities. It is generally accepted that the purpose of an assessment and the particular behaviour under investigation determine to a great extent both the content and the form of an assessment procedure. However, there are a number of basic principles that hold for all such procedures.

As will be seen, these are for the most part the same principles as those that underlie psychological tests in general, and as such will be largely familiar to most practising therapists. Nevertheless, they are outlined here partly because we do not want to restrict the readership to speech and language therapists and, equally importantly, because their relative weight might be different in assessment procedures that are specifically designed to evaluate communicative effectiveness.

Commonly accepted wisdom says that any test, whether a paper and pencil one or an oral interview, must have two characteristics, namely reliability and validity. These are absolutely crucial for the test to function as an appropriate instrument.

Validity

In general terms, the validity of a test is a reflection of the degree to which it actually measures what it was designed to measure and nothing else. There are several different kinds of validity:

1. Face validity – this relates to the types of task contained in a test. Measures of face validity indicate the extent to which a test looks as if it measures what it is supposed to. In terms of communicative ability, oral interviews, for example, have a high face validity because they are supposed to resemble real life situations, whereas picture descriptions and naming tasks have a low face validity. Neither of them are activities people often engage in.
2. Content validity – this relates to the representativeness of tasks or items included in the test. In view of what has been said about communication, one of the most formidable challenges for a communication assessment is to capture the overwhelming complexity of

communication behaviour. As so many different factors interact it is particularly difficult to design tasks which can take them all into account. Besides, the occurrence of a particular communicative act depends on many external conditions. The question is whether it is necessary and possible to create contexts for all types of behaviour.

3. Predictive validity – this is a measure of the extent to which a test has predictive value. This requirement is also problematic in view of the variety of factors that influence how a person communicates.

4. Construct validity – this is a reflection of the extent to which the test reflects the tenets of a particular theory. At present there are no comprehensive theories that allow us to systematically correlate the form communication takes with the many different parameters listed under the components of communication. In the absence of such theories we have to be satisfied with merely taking those components into account.

5. Concurrent validity – this relates to how closely the scores of a test relate to some other test. This is the most difficult to achieve because so few tests actually measure the same behaviour in comparable ways.

If the aim is to arrive at a realistic way of assessing communicative abilities the most important types of validity are content validity, face validity and predictive validity.

Reliability

This requirement is concerned with the extent to which tests are capable of producing consistent results when they are administered under similar conditions. Reliability can also be subdivided into several types:

1. Rater reliability – this can be either intra-rater or inter-rater reliability. In the first, a test is reliable if on subsequent scoring by the same rater identical or at least similar scores are achieved, and in the second case where identical or similar scores are achieved by two separate raters. Even where communicative abilities are scorable it is unlikely that two testers would ever achieve identical scoring, especially where the evaluation requires the tester to exercise individual judgement. As has already been pointed out, individual judgements are inevitable and even necessary (Ingram, 1985) in judging communicative behaviour. However, there is evidence in the literature on second language learning that subjectivity can be greatly reduced by training (Clark, 1983; Shohamy, 1983) There is also evidence from the learning disabilities field that inter-rater reliability can be achieved when assessing certain aspects of communication. Concerns about the reliability of carers' judgements were investigated by van der Gaag (1989). The study analysed joint assessments

made by 384 carers and 66 speech and language therapists using the Communication Assessment Profile (CASP) (see Chapter 4 for a description of this assessment). The mean level of agreement between the two groups who had assessed the same clients at different times was 0.68 ($p<0.001$) so van der Gaag concluded that these carers were able to make reliable judgements when given a structured assessment with which to work.

2. Item reliability – this relates to the extent to which single items can contribute to the total score. This is normally a very useful measure when testing populations, and it reflects the extent to which test items consistently rank people in the same way. In view of the complexity of communicative behaviour, this requirement poses a particularly difficult challenge to assessment procedures aiming at an evaluation of global communicative behaviour. It inevitably relates back to the requirement of content validity, in particular to the need for a representative sample. At the moment, no conclusive evidence exists as to the precise contribution of particular behaviours on overall communicative effectiveness. A great deal of research is needed in order to establish predictive tendencies.

3. Test–retest reliability – as the term indicates, this measure relates to the similarity or otherwise of scores achieved on a second testing. As communicative situations vary so much, the value of this particular measure may not be of great importance in assessing communicative ability, unless of course identical conditions can be artificially constructed.

Special Needs for Learning-disabled Adults

There are a number of additional considerations which have to do with the practicalities of administering assessment procedures in a 'clinical'-type setting. What are the practical considerations specific to this group of individuals?

In the last few years, over 1000 professionals in the UK have attended workshops on communication assessment led by one of the present authors and attended by speech and language therapists and carers. One of the aims was to examine communication assessment from a multidisciplinary perspective. This included looking in some detail at the difficulties of assessing the communication skills of people with learning disabilities. Some of what follows is based upon the work undertaken by these groups. Despite the wide-ranging background and experience found in each group, a remarkably cohesive account of the salient problems of assessment emerged. They have been summarised under four headings:

1. Tool/material-related problems.
2. Staff-related problems.

3. Client-related problems.
4. Environment-related problems.

Tools-related problems

Not enough time to assess

Almost all the groups discussed the problem of lack of time for assessment. It was generally felt that it was impossible to justify spending so much time on assessment when there were so many clients to deal with. This is a concern often expressed by speech and language therapists in general, and it is an important concern. Given the limited amount of time and resources, the length of an assessment procedure must be carefully monitored. However, the question of time spent on assessment in relation to time spent in intervention merits some discussion. Although it is rarely articulated, there seems to be a belief among some speech and language therapists that assessment is a preliminary and sometimes marginalised job that needs to be over and done with as quickly as possible before the serious work of intervention can begin. It is a little like tidying up one's desk before one can settle down to doing any real work. This kind of attitude misses two important points. One is that assessment is not a one-off activity at the beginning of an intervention programme. On the contrary, it must be an ongoing part of the intervention; indeed, the possibility and the necessity of it inevitably emerge with each intervention task a client embarks upon. The second point is that, provided the rationale is clear, spending 'so much time' on assessment is more than likely to save time in intervention and is almost guaranteed to be more effective than intervention based upon superficial assessment. Weak assessment leads to weak intervention which, in turn, leads to weak results.

Inappropriate assessments

A large number of the available assessment materials were not considered by the group participants to be at all appropriate to people with learning disabilities. The reasons for this lie primarily in the enormous range of ages and abilities of people with learning disabilities, but also in the practice of administering tests designed for children with language difficulties, or for aphasic adults (Cottam, 1986; Dormandy and van der Gaag, 1989).

Assessments focus on the negative

Tests were frequently considered to focus on the negative aspects of a client's communication. As we have already discussed, this is not an inevitable property of tests. Much depends upon the interpretation of test results. However, what does seem to be of great importance for all tests or assessment procedures of any kind is the need to bear in mind the role of the affective factors in testing. These include test anxiety. Scott and Madsen (1983) suggest that 'test anxious...individuals fail to perform up to capacity on tests of intelligence, aptitude and short term memory'. Clearly, tests should be aimed at what clients know rather than what their weaknesses are in the test environment.

Staff-related problems

1. Both carers and speech and language therapists who took part in the workshops thought that one of the overriding problems in communication assessment was that speech and language therapy expertise was frequently not available or could not be offered.
2. 'Professionalism' among therapists was one of the criticisms made by the carers, some of whom felt that speech and language therapists often used jargon and did not do enough to share information with them.
3. Another concern was the lack of appropriate training, or too little training, for carers.
4. Some speech and language therapists felt that carers' expectations of clients were sometimes too low and that, as a result, it was often difficult to motivate carers to become involved in intervention.

Client-related problems

The difficulties of accurately assessing people with learning disabilities are well documented by Morse (1988). In recent years, some of the proponents of normalisation theory have argued that any kind of assessment contravenes the principle that adults with learning disabilities should be treated with the same degree of respect as any other human being. Assessment, they argue, is patronising and devalues the people being assessed by placing them in a submissive and passive role (Brechin and Swain, 1988). In order to avoid the risk of disadvantaging the person, the factors likely to influence their response to an assessment situation must be recognised (Morse, 1988). These include:

1. The individual's knowledge and experience of the vocabulary used in the assessment of vocabulary. In the course of assessing a child or aphasic adult's language abilities, it is customary to administer a standardised vocabulary test. The standardisation has normally been carried out on similar populations of normally speaking children or adults. Adults with learning disabilities have frequently been compared with either of these two groups, neither of which are relevant (Dormandy and van der Gaag, 1989). We argue that it would be

much more appropriate to design individually based vocabulary assessments in place of these more general vocabulary tests.

2. The audibility of the speaker. This may seem all too obvious, but adults with learning disabilities are frequently assessed in noisy rooms, where they cannot hear the assessor properly.

3. The listener's auditory perception and discrimination skills. Nolan et al. (1980) highlight the relatively high incidence of hearing impairment among adults with learning disabilities. Assessors need to be aware of this when using an assessment that relies heavily on auditory cues, for example, a picture pointing task.

4. The rate at which materials are presented. There is evidence that some people with learning disabilities may have a slow response to visual or auditory prompts. For example, Merrill (1985) looked at the language processing skills of a group of learning-disabled people. He found that the group differed from their control counterparts not so much in their ability to process semantics, but in the speed at which they were able to do this.

5. The listener's interest in the materials. This relates very closely to the familiarity factor outlined in 1 above. If the materials presented are inappropriate or of no interest to the individual, then this will influence how he or she responds. This particular problem is not specific to adults with learning disabilities but it is often ignored in this context because standardised tests, when they are used, do not allow flexibility in materials and content.

6. The listener's cognitive abilities. The relationship between language and cognitive skills is a complex one. An individual's knowledge of the world greatly influences what he or she can communicate about and how. The precise nature of the relationship between language and cognition remains unknown, perhaps more so among adults, where the influence of age and experience may have a compounding effect on both cognitive and linguistic skills (van der Gaag, 1985). The great variability of cognitive abilities in people with learning disabilities also makes predictions from one behaviour to another more problematic.

7. Visual perception. This is another area where a person with a learning disability and physical disability can face considerable obstacles in an assessment setting. Poor visual skills may well prevent him or her from responding consistently or correctly on picture pointing or picture naming tasks (Yeates, 1980).

8. Restricted physical movements. Over one-third of intellectually disabled people have some form of physical disability. The physically disabled person may well be able to understand the task, but may not be able to respond appropriately.

Morse (1988) observed that the majority of standardised measures demand a basic level of motor control, visual perceptual ability and auditory processing skills which the learning-disabled individual may not have at his or her command. If we are trying to measure linguistic abilities, understanding and use of language, then we must acknowledge the influence of these peripheral processes and functions on the central language processes. We must know what they are and how they may be influencing the individual's communication.

9. The listener–speaker relationship. We noted earlier the vital importance of this factor for communication in general. It gains special significance in relation to adults with learning disabilities. Davies and Mehan (1988) found marked differences in professionals' versus carers' perceptions of a severely communication-disabled woman. The professionals judged her communicative ability to be at a much lower level than her carers did. Davies and Mehan conclude that the degree of familiarity and rapport that exists between speaker and listener will have a marked influence on the way an individual's communication is assessed. It may therefore be necessary to investigate communicative function in a variety of settings with a variety of communicative partners.

10. Emotional factors, past experiences, temperament and personal characteristics. Linked with the above are the personality factors that inevitably influence the assessment procedure. If the individual being tested has experienced a sense of failure in the past, he or she may, quite justifiably, be reluctant to cooperate. Such individuals may equally be inclined to try and over-compensate for their difficulty, wanting to succeed in everything while being aware that they cannot. This can lead to perseveration, or to a delayed response to a request, or to attempts to change the subject.

Environment-related problems

Recording the right information in the right context

The difficulty of recording communication in context was mentioned by many of the participants at the communication assessment workshops. They frequently asked: 'How do we look at communication behaviour in a way that is relevant'? 'How do we record information about a client's communication when he appears to communicate differently in different contexts?' These are important questions, which this book hopes to address in some measure at least. We have already observed that what is relevant to one population may not be for another. In addition, one-off testing situations may be particularly problematic for adults, for the reasons outlined above. It goes without saying that assessment should be carried out at a time that is convenient to the individual; if it is not, then this may further bias the outcome of the assessment.

Discrepancies between assessors

Another environment-related problem mentioned at the communication assessment workshops was the fact that clients communicate differently in different settings, which can mean that there is a discrepancy between different assessors' views of the individual's ability. This is true of all of us – it is not peculiar to adults with learning disabilities. The same extroverted and loquacious student one meets in the corridor outside the lecture theatre turns into a reticent mute when asked a question a few minutes later in the course of the lecture.

The Content of Communication Assessment

The content of a communication assessment also needs to be dictated by the components of communication. As we have seen, this is a vast and complicated area and the problem lies in trying to pare it down in such a way that meaningful information can be gained about a client's communication abilities (Davies and Wilcox, 1983). A choice must be made as to whether the assessment should aim at evaluating the total 'communicative behaviour', or focus on one component of it. Both may be necessary, but at different times. It is as important to gain an overall picture as it is to identify the relative contribution of each component to the whole.

Apart from assessing the linguistic abilities of clients whenever this is appropriate, other abilities which can be influenced by context, such as paralinguistic, non-linguistic and conversational abilities, will need to be examined. For example, we need to examine the comprehension and production of prosodic features which are used to express emotion; the ability to use non-verbal skills both to interpret messages and to convey them in order to augment or replace verbal communication; the use of turn taking; the ability to initiate, sustain and terminate a communicative event; and sensitivity to the communicative partner's needs and abilities. Individuals with communication difficulties quite often develop idiosyncratic verbal and non-verbal behaviours, often referred to as compensatory strategies. The communicative effectiveness of these need also to be considered.

What Methods of Assessment Are Currently Being Used?

There are a number of methods used to assess communication skills in adults with learning disabilities:

1. IQ tests.
2. Standardised language assessments.

3. Behavioural checklists.
4. Functional communication checklists.
5. Observational assessments.
6. Profiling.

IQ tests

IQ tests carry a qualification restriction and are usually administered by psychologists. They examine verbal and non-verbal skills. Performance on each item of the test is scored and then compared with a normal distribution of scores, frequently providing cross-comparisons between chronological age, mental age and IQ score and a classification ('severe–mild mental handicap). The value of IQ tests has been questioned, particularly as far as validity is concerned (Morse, 1988).The content validity of IQ tests is widely felt to be suspect, and according to Ingram (1976),' the essential truth about nearly all kinds of tests is that the only theory they are based on is test construction theory, which is a kind of applied statistics. Current intelligence tests are not based on any coherent or explicit cognitive theory.' In other words, the construct validity of IQ tests may be in question. IQ tests are rarely used in the UK or the USA with learning-disabled adults, essentially because they fail to produce information that is relevant to intervention (Edgerton, 1984; Coolidge et al., 1986).

Standardised language assessments

The standardised language assessment was until relatively recently the speech and language therapist's most widely used method of assessment, in both the USA and the UK (Pickett and Flynn, 1983; Cottam, 1986; Calculator and Bedrosian, 1988).

This method involves using a standard set of materials in order to assess a specific range of communicative abilities in a one-off, one-to-one context. It requires the individual being assessed to work through a series of tasks in which the response to each task will be judged as either correct or incorrect. The responses are recorded and scored, and the total score is compared with a norm or standard. There are three essential properties of standardised assessments: they are norm referenced, they are discrete point tests and they are indirect tests of ability in specific areas.

Norm referencing

Traditionally, speech and language therapists, like other professionals working in the field, have used standardised assessments which have been norm referenced on a particular population. These assessments provide norms of communication behaviour based on a population sample's performance on a particular range of tasks. Norm-referenced tests are used in the identification of delay or deficit, that is, to provide a fairly gross indication of the child's or adult's level of ability, on an intelligence or developmental scale, and to say something about the degree of delay or deficit present. Because these tests provide normative comparisons, they are also used as guidelines for the educational placement of children.

Discrete point tests

A common characteristic of standardised language assessments is that language is seen as consisting of separate, distinct categories, and test items are designed to assess one particular such category. A number of individual items of language or behaviour are selected for testing production or comprehension. This, it is assumed, can provide an accurate estimate as to an individual's global behaviour. This approach is referred to as discrete point testing. The criteria for selecting these discrete items can be quite ad hoc. Test items are often chosen simply on the intuition and experience of the examiner. Often the examiner's intuition is assisted by 'tradition', although the forms endorsed by 'tradition' are often equally ad hoc and intuitive (Ingram, 1985).

A second criterion for selecting an item for a standardised test has a more practical base. Some items are easier to elicit or to present for comprehension than others, given the limited range of materials normally available in the clinical context. Presumably this is why, for example, the assessment of adjectives is normally restricted to colour, shape and size, both in child and adult assessments.

Ease of scoring is also an important consideration in selecting test items. Norm-referenced standardised tests tend to concentrate upon behaviours which are measurable in numeric terms, and which supposedly provide an index for normal development, but which are not necessarily 'crucial behaviours' (i.e. those without which subsequent development will not occur). In addition to this scorability requirement, the need to control all variables other than the specific test items imposes further constraints on the choice of items selected for testing.

Indirect tests of ability in certain areas

It follows partly from being discrete point tests that standardised tests are indirect tests of ability in certain areas. The communicative behaviours required by them hardly ever occur in actual communicative situations. Even if a task is designed so that it represents a real-life situation, it is not necessarily the case that the behaviour elicited in the test context reflects the way an individual would act in such a situation.

So what can standardised assessments tell us? There are a number of reasons why standardised tests have been so popular. Some of these are real, some are imaginary in the context of communication at least. The following are some of the positive characteristics that have been put forward. Standardised tests provide the assessor with:

1. A quantitative measure of the individual's performance on certain set tasks.
2. A measure of change over time, that is, a yardstick against which any subsequent progress can be measured, at least as far as performance on these tasks is concerned.
3. A baseline of abilities upon which to begin intervention.
4. A set route to identifying the individual's communication problems.
5. A comparison with the norm.
6. A structure which is all-inclusive, and does not rely upon the assessor's memory for what should be assessed.

It may be helpful at this stage to look more closely at a specific standardised language test. The Carrow Test of Auditory Comprehension is just one example of a standardised test which concurs with the characteristics outlined above (Carrow, 1973). This test consists of 101 sets of three pictures, each testing the understanding of a particular syntactic structure. The assessor gives the verbal cue, and the individual being tested must point to the picture that matches the verbal cue. The Carrow Test of Auditory Comprehension purports to measure understanding of syntactic structures on four levels:

1. Word categories: nouns, verbs, adjectives, interrogatives, demonstratives.
2. Morphological constructions: noun + '-er'; verb + '-er'; noun + '-er' (masculine suffix) 'fisherman'; adjective + '-er/est' 'smallest'; noun + '-ist' 'cyclist'.
3. Grammatical categories: gender + number; pronoun: 'he, she, they'; number + '-s'; tense; status: verb 'the girl is drawing'.
4. Syntactic structure: imperatives; predication: noun verb agreement; complementation; modification; coordination.

What information will this test give about the individual being tested? It will give information about his or her ability to understand a number of different linguistic forms in the absence of contextual or other cues to meaning. Like most other standardised measures, it examines this and only this aspect of communicative competence. It makes no assessment of how the individual is using language in context. The choice of linguistic items must of necessity be ad hoc. It is certainly not grounded in current linguistic theory. In the word level categories all the nouns are represented by objects and all the verbs are represented by 'doing' words. A noun is not a noun because it stands for objects, but because it occupies specific positions in sentences, and can take specific affixes. Verbs are also defined in terms of their distribution, and so are all the other word categories. Unless words are used in sentences it is often impossible to tell what category they belong to. For example, the word 'jump' is a verb in one context, for example, 'the horses jump over the fence', but it is a noun in another, e.g. 'I did not see their jump'. Because of this, the word category part of the test is a simple vocabulary test and not a test of grammar at all. The same can be said about the subtest which looks at 'morphological construction'. Four out of the five types of constructions are word formation types and only one of them is grammatical. In addition, four out of the five have the form '-er'. Someone being tested could well fail these items for phonological rather than either grammatical or lexical reasons. There are problems with the other subtests, which make any prediction on the basis of the items contained in the test extremely suspect. In short, this test fails on most measures of validity.

It is not, of course, a prerequisite of standardised tests that they should contain items that disregard current linguistic theories, but unfortunately a very large number of the tests used in routine speech and language therapy assessment do. The problem of testing out of context, however, is shared by all of these tests. They are all therefore questionable as far as content validity, and therefore predictive validity, is concerned. In addition, these tests do not provide information which can form the basis of intervention strategies. Standardised tests as used in psychological testing were, in fact, never intended to be used as therapeutic tools. As these tests provide normative comparisons, and are designed to measure individual differences, their best use is for the educational placement of children, or possibly for screening purposes where populations need to be classified into groups. Apart from the inherent shortcomings of these tests as far as intervention is concerned, there really is little purpose in using them to evaluate an individual's communicative behaviour, just as there is no need for standardised assessments for driving tests. It does not matter how much one candidate's driving ability compares to another's. What matters is whether she or he can safely drive a car from A to B. Even here, context will influence outcome. The standard of driving required in the Kalahari desert will be very different from that required in Rome or New York.

One of the advantages claimed for standardised tests was that they provided the assessor with a baseline measure of behaviour. They do achieve this, but only on the test items contained in the test. As no realistic predictions can be based on these, the value of this baseline is not great.

As for the claimed advantage that these tests are all-inclusive and therefore do not rely on the assessor's memory for what should be assessed, it must be remembered that the range of behaviours they measure is very limited. An assessor who is satisfied with what a discrete point standardised test is capable of measuring must realise that she or he is not measuring 'communication'. The reasons for the limitations are inherent in these tests and, as Kiernan and Jones (1982) have suggested, there is a danger that this kind of approach can give more attention to the less than crucial items. Take this example from O'Connor's (1989) examination of an autistic child:

> Michael has no speech at all and although diagnosed as autistic clearly has a much more complex range of disabilities...On one occasion we measured Michael's IQ on the Matrices...[Raven's Matrices], a test supposedly of culture free intelligence. He scored well above normal...Later we measured him on the Columbia – an 'odd one out' test. This test contains Matrice like spatial oddity tests but also tests depending on knowledge of daily life events. Michael's IQ was found to be about 70.

These kinds of discrepancies are well documented in the literature on norm-referenced testing (Naglieri, 1985; Merrill, 1985; Morse, 1988).

One thing that can be said about standardised tests is that they all do well in relation to the various criteria of reliability. However, as has been pointed out, absolute reliability is probably neither realistic nor indeed a desirable criterion for evaluating human behaviour.

Criterion referencing

In contrast to norm-referenced tests, criterion-referenced assessments are concerned with an individual's ability to achieve certain targets in order to function adequately in his or her environment (Kiernan and Jones, 1982). In other words, criterion-referenced tests are not concerned with an individual's performance relative to others, but with describing the individual's abilities within a particular skill area. In most instances, this information is directly relevant to intervention planning. This type of assessment is not necessarily dependent on a one-off assessment of the individual's abilities; it may rely on several observations at different times. According to Glaser and Nitko (1971) a criterion-referenced test is one that is 'deliberately constructed to give measurements that are directly related to performance standards'. Criterion referencing looks at the pattern of performance, the content of performance as opposed to the test score. Those who advocate the use of criterion-referenced assessment do so for several reasons:

1. Criterion-referenced tests assess the individual only in relation to himself or herself, his or her strengths, needs, and ability to function.
2. It provides information relevant to intervention.
3. It reduces the likelihood that an individual's skills or abilities will be

judged on the basis of a one-off assessment from which a numeric score is derived.

According to Beaumeister (1968), people with learning disabilities may be variable in their responses, particularly in demand situations. Any single observation of performance is therefore likely to result in an underestimate of the learning-disabled person's optimal level. Using criterion-referenced assessment will, in part, avoid this description of behaviour only in terms of the 'level of performance' concept.

Goodstein (1982) also warns against placing too much store by criterion-referenced tests. He points out that errors can be made just as they are in norm-referenced testing – the instrument is only ever as good as its user. Both Popham (1981) and Kiernan and Jones (1982) suggest that the fundamental difference between criterion-referenced and norm-referenced tests lies in the manner in which the individual performance is interpreted. It is possible to use a norm-referenced test with a criterion-referenced approach, i.e. where the norm is the criterion. Instead of focusing on the scores achieved the emphasis is on how the individual performs on each item, and looking for patterns in his or her performance. This approach is capable of providing the assessor with more qualitative information which, in turn, is more useful and serves more purpose in planning intervention strategies.

Behavioural checklists

Checklists of general ability are used extensively in the UK and in the USA. In Britain, Gunzburg's Progress Assessment Charts (PAC), devised in the 1960s, began a tradition of descriptive checklisting of behaviours, none of which were norm referenced to either a child or an adult population. More recent checklists of this kind include the Copewell Checklist (Whelan and Speake, 1974), the Hampshire Assessment for Living with Others (Shackleton Bailey, 1983), and Pathways to Independence (Jeffree and Cheseldine, 1986).

These checklists provide the assessor with a list of behaviours against which she or he can compare the abilities of the client. In most instances, these checklists require the assessor to make a subjective evaluation based on day to day observations. Some offer guidelines on how to elicit certain behaviours, but without the constraints imposed by the standardised one-off assessment. These assessments are usually carried out by the client's carer. They can obviously offer only a limited amount of information on communication skills, as they cover all aspects of behaviour from knowledge of local transport facilities to sexual awareness. The breadth of coverage is at the cost of depth.

In the USA, where the tradition of standardised assessment is probably much stronger than it is in the UK, a number of checklists have been norm referenced. These include the Vineland Social Maturity

Scales (Doll (1935, 1990) , which was standardised on a 'normal' adult population, and the Adaptive Behaviour Scales (Nihira et al., 1975), which was standardised on learning-disabled adults.

The advantage of these checklists is that they are not domain specific, and so provide a general picture of the individual's abilities. The disadvantage is that they are frequently too superficial to form the basis of any communication intervention.

Checklists of functional communication

Similar to checklists of general ability, these assessments provide the assessor with a list of communicative functions against which he or she can compare the client's communication skills. The Functional Communication Profile (Sarno, 1969), and the recently revised Edinburgh Functional Communication Profile (Skinner et al., 1984, 1990) are two of the most widely used examples. However, checklists such as these purport to measure only communicative function. They cannot give a comprehensive view of the individual's communicative effectiveness because they make no analysis of linguistic competence. They are therefore frequently used in conjunction with other measures.

Ethnographic assessment

Ethnography, or the study of people in naturalistic settings, is an approach which has its roots in anthropology and sociology (see Chapter 9). Its application to the lives of people with learning disabilities was pioneered by Edgerton and his colleagues in California (Edgerton, 1967). Edgerton's basic premise was that a true understanding of the lives of people with disabilities can only come from the study of their natural life experiences, rather than from experiences contrived to elicit certain behaviours. This approach, unlike the others outlined above, relies upon long-term and often intense involvement in the lives of the people who are being assessed (Edgerton, 1967; Turner et al., 1984). In many instances, assessors share in the lives of the people they are assessing over several months or years, and make detailed analyses of audio and video tapes of their interactions. This method has provided a great deal of information on the communicative abilities of adults with learning disabilities. Unfortunately, the resources required are often considerable, and consequently there are few centres that use Edgerton's approach in quite this way. However, a number of therapists are using very similar methods which are firmly rooted in the ethnographic tradition, even though they do not involve the same degree of time commitment. Bedrosian (1982), for example, describes a sociolinguistic approach to assessing communication skills. This involves recording the individual in conversation in a number of naturalistic settings for a specified time period (perhaps about 20 minutes), and then examining the interactions using a detailed system of conversational analysis. Examples of this approach are described in detail by Bedrosian and Prutting (1978), Owings and MacManus (1980) and Bedrosian (1988).

Another example of ethnographic methods in use in the USA comes from Brown et al. (1979), who devised an ecological assessment procedure known as the Ecological and Student Repertoire Inventory (ESRI). This method requires all the assessments to be carried out in the context of whatever skill is being taught at the time. The first stage of the assessment is to determine exactly what skills are required by an individual without disabilities operating in the same context. This constitutes establishing the 'ecological inventory' of skills. The second stage involves assessing the skills of the individual, or 'student' (known as the'student' inventory), in relation to the ecological inventory. The final stage is to determine ways and means of matching the two inventories.

If, for example, one were looking at the skills required to stack canned food in a supermarket, the first stage of the ESRI process would be to identify what skills were necessary to do the job. These would include finding the appropriate shelves in the supermarket, arranging the cans already on the shelves to make room for more cans, taking the new cans out of the box and arranging them on the shelves, taking the cans that do not fit on the shelves back to the storeroom, and disposing of any empty boxes. The final stage in this example would be to devise the best ways of teaching each skill to the student until a match between the ecological inventory and the student inventory could be made. The ESRI process is very detailed, and can work for mechanistic skills such as the one described above. Its value for communication assessment and intervention is problematic, in that it is not always clear what processes must take place in order to achieve success as a communicator.

In Britain, the ethnographic approach to assessment is probably less well known among speech and language therapists. It does, however, manifest itself in the use of audio and video recordings of naturally occurring conversations, or rather as natural as they can be under such circumstances. The measurement of interactional styles and communicative functions has gradually become more precise (Dewart and Summers, 1989) as clinicians become more focused on this area. (For a more detailed discussion of ethnography and its contribution to the field, see Chapter 9.)

Profiling

Somewhere between the overly rigorous standardised tests and the naturalistic observations fall the various linguistic and communication profiles that have been developed in the last two decades. According to Crystal, 'a linguistic profile is a principled description of just those features of a person's use of language which enable him to be identified for a specific purpose' (Crystal, 1982). Comparing profiles to tests he lists three main advantages:

1. Profiles are more flexible and comprehensive than tests.
2. Profiles 'try to focus attention on remedial paths in a systematic and theoretically motivated way'.
3. Whereas test scores are summaries of individual achievements, profiles allow a more subjective evaluation of a whole range of findings.

Following Crystal's purely linguistic profiles, a number of communication profiles appeared of which perhaps Prutting and Kirchner's Pragmatic Protocol is the probably one of the best known in speech and language therapy clinics (Prutting and Kirchner, 1983). Although it is not specifically aimed at adults with learning disabilities, it contains largely the same type of parameters that are seen as important in functional communication assessments in general. These constitute a set of pragmatic paralinguistic and non-linguistic behaviours which normally accompany verbal communication, such as the organisation of conversations, body language and quality of delivery. The behaviours are listed and evaluated according to appropriateness or otherwise, rather than scored numerically. The Pragmatic Protocol's strengths and shortcomings are very similar to those communication profiles that have been developed for adults with learning disabilities, and which are described in the following chapter. We therefore postpone our comments regarding its usefulness until the end of the next chapter.

Chapter 4
Recent Developments in Communication Assessment and Intervention

In 1987, Scott et al. described how the role of the speech and language therapist working with adults with learning disabilities was undergoing considerable change. They suggested that 'traditional ' one-to-one speech therapy with individual clients was no longer appropriate in the context of day and residential services to adults. They described how more and more therapists were becoming involved in teaching and training carers, and in delivering 'indirect' therapy via carers. This view had already been put forward by a number of authors in the USA and the UK, including Guyette (1978), Halle et al. (1988), Owings and Guyette (1982), Stansfield (1982), McCartney et al. (1984), Elstob (1986) and Kersner (1987).

The emergence of this model is likely to be attributable to a number of influences; the first is the realisation that changes in communication skills are more likely to generalise from the therapeutic context when the client's communicative environment is taken into account (Guyette, 1978; Halle et al., 1988; Bedrosian, 1988; Leudar, 1988; van der Gaag, 1989; Hurst Brown and Keens, 1990; Jones, 1990). This necessitates the involvement of carers in the therapeutic process; indeed, it makes their contribution essential to the success of speech therapy intervention. It also takes communication assessment out of the clinical setting and into the naturalistic contexts in which individuals communicate. Halle (1988), for example, describes an assessment and intervention approach that concentrates on assessing comunication skills in the context of everyday life and activities, and on assessing the 'language requirements' of particular settings. This involves asking questions like 'What language skills does the individual need to have in order to be a successful communicator in this particular setting?' Similarly, Bedrosian has developed an assessment process that looks at discourse behaviours such as turn taking, topic initations and repair, degree of conversational control, politeness and non-verbal behaviour as they are used with different individuals in different contexts. Calculator and Bedrosian (1988) summarise these approaches to communication assessment as 'an informal examination of communicative performance in a variety of natural contexts' (p.342). The emphasis is on decribing the individual's strengths and weaknesses in relation to his unique communicative and social setting, rather than making comparisons with any norms or standards.

A second major influence is the recognition that there are not enough speech and language therapists to meet the demand for speech therapy expertise among this population (Cottam, 1986; Enderby and Davies, 1989). Very few speech therapy services have the resources to deliver therapy on a one to one basis in any average-sized day centre, where the estimated percentage of adults with an identifiable communication difficulty may be as high as 89% (Noble, 1990).

A third influence we would suggest represents a less well founded argument. Many speech and language therapists now assert that the so-called linguistic aspects of language are not relevant to intervention with adults with learning disabilities. This view arises from some major misconceptions about the contribution of linguistics to communication assessment and intervention techniques. For example, the most pervasive view is that speech therapy intervention can only modify the pragmatic component of language, and can do little in the area of language structure. There is some evidence that the pragmatic component of language may, at least superficially, be more strongly influenced by the communication environment than other components (Curtiss and Yamada, 1980; Sabsay and Platt, 1984; van der Gaag, 1989). This does not, however, mean that the linguistic aspects of language should be ignored altogether. There is also some evidence that pragmatic aspects of language use have a role in shaping the formal aspects of language (Gazdar and Levinson, 1979, 1983; Bates and McWhinney, 1982). It may well be true that the majority of current linguistic models familiar to speech and language therapists are not approprate. This is partly due to the models themselves, in that they tend not to pay enough attention to the functional aspects of language (Bedrosian, 1988), but concentrate on the individual subsystems of language such as phonology, syntax or vocabulary in isolation, without providing an overview of how language works, or how it is used to communicate. For example, sections of available standardised tests that look at the linguistic components of language are theoretically unsound and fragmentary. In addition to this, it may be that many speech and language therapists do not feel confident enough to implement linguistically based strategies, despite the fact that linguistics has been part of speech therapy training for the last 15 years or so.

In the light of these influences it is not surprising that the most recently produced communication assessments for adults with learning disabilities are quite different in form and emphasis from the more 'traditional' speech therapy assessment procedures. This chapter describes four such assessments devised and produced in the UK during the last 5 years. A discussion of their relative strengths and weaknesses follows towards the end of the chapter.

Communication Assessment Profile (van der Gaag, 1988)

The Communication Assessment Profile (CASP) has been described as a 'functional screening assessment...with a strong leaning towards community relevance' (Cheseldine, 1990). It was designed for use with adults with learning disabilities at a time when there were no other published communication assessments for this population in the UK. It is primarily for use with adults with severe to mild learning disabilities. It is a descriptive assessment, which combines a number of different methods of assessment in one 'package': formal and informal observations, structured language tasks, checklists of communicative function, elicited conversation. The CASP is based upon the premise that the carer and the speech and language therapist should have equal status in the assessment procedure, and that both undertake a specific role within it.

The profile is divided into three parts. The first is completed by the client's carer or 'keyworker' , that is, the individual who is in contact with the client on a day to day basis. The second part is completed by the speech and language therapist, and the final part is completed by both carer and therapist. Using this framework, the CASP offers a way of assessing the client's understanding and expression of language, his or her ability to use this knowledge in everyday activities, and the 'communicative demands' that are made on him or her.

The theoretical basis for CASP

CASP as an asset-based approach

The first and most important of the three theoretical underpinnings of CASP is that it is an asset-based assessment. This distinguishes it from many other assessments which have been used in the past with people with learning disabilities, and which are 'deficit based'. These assessments compare the person being assessed with some norm or standard which is not relevant to an adult with a learning disability, for example a population of children, or adults with dysphasia. An asset-based assessment is one that seeks to describe the person's abilities, rather than focus on what he or she cannot do.

CASP as an ecological approach

The second theoretical underpinning is that CASP follows an ecological approach to assessment. Its primary concern is with the functional aspects of language and communication, how language works in practice for a particular person (Owings and Guyette, 1982; Landesman Dwyer and Knowles, 1987; Murphy, 1987; van der Gaag, 1988; Hurst Brown and Keens, 1990; Jones, 1990; Hitchins and Spence, 1991). Owings and Guyette argued that the 'communication demands placed on an individual by his environment should provide the basis for any intervention programme'. They describe this as 'environment–ability matching', as opposed to 'age–ability' matching. In environment–ability matching the client's abilities are examined in relation to his or her communication environment. In age–ability matching, the client's abilities are examined in relation to a developmental standard or norm.

Formalising the role of the carer

The notion of environment–ability matching provides the central rationale for involving carers in the assessment process. In order to gain a truly representative picture of the client's communication skills in context, the individual who knows the client well *must* be involved in describing his or her abilities. A further discussion of involving carers is described by van der Gaag (1989). Collaboration of this kind serves three purposes:

1. Personal and professional relationships can be developed through understanding the other's perspective on assessment.
2. Combining objective and subjective assessments by different individuals, ascribing equal value to all those involved. The majority of widely used communication assessments do not involve the carer until after formal assessments have been completed by the professional. The carer's subjective views are sought and taken into consideration, but their role is not formalised.
3. The third 'purpose' in collaborative assessment is one which Warnock (1979) discussed, and which the UK Community Care Bill and the Childrens Act (1989) depend upon. It is simply that equal status should be ascribed to all those involved in the assessment process. For many years the word of the professional has been gospel, taking precedence over the opinions of carers. There is now a recognition that carers, or 'significant others', have equally important contributions to make, and that they should be seen as active not passive members of the team, contributors to, not just recipients of, information.

Language and communication

The CASP is based upon the view that communication is dependent upon two factors, a successful interaction between the different levels or subcomponents of language such as phonology, syntax, semantics and pragmatics; and a successful interaction between the individual's language skills and his 'communication environment'. This refers to the opportunities individuals have to use their communication skills, and the demands that are made upon them to communicate (Owings and Guyette 1982).

In addition, van der Gaag (1989) describes communicative competence as an interaction between an individual's linguistic competence (phonology, syntax, and semantics), his or her pragmatic competence, (Price Williams and Sabsay, 1979) and the communication environment (Guyette,1978). Any communication assessment must incorporate a measure of all of these elements.

Description of CASP

CASP is divided into three parts. Each of these is described in some detail below.

Carer's assessment

The carer's assessment is a questionnaire which is completed by the client's carer, keyworker or equivalent – someone who knows the client well on a day to day basis.

The first section is a checklist of communicative functions, based upon the work of Chapman (1972) and Miller (1978). They provided the following summary of the functional uses of language: giving information, initiating a conversation, asking questions, responding to questions, describing events and feelings, telling jokes and stories. In the carer's assessment, each of these functional uses of language is presented to the carer as a question to which he or she has to respond positively or negatively; for example. initiating a conversation:
Q: Does the client ever begin a conversation with you?

These communicative functions are also assessed by the speech and language therapist.

The second section of the assessment is designed to record information about the client's communication environment: his or her interests, hobbies, responsibilities, educational interests and home circumstances where relevant, for example, siblings, friendships, holidays, regular social events etc.

Therapist's assessment

This part of CASP is completed by the speech and language therapist. It comprises eight subsections and an Appendix, each of which allows the therapist to look at the different subcomponents of language outlined above. These are examined using a variety of assessment methods.

Event knowledge

The aim of this section is to establish some rapport with the client, and to begin to assess his or her use of communication in a conversational context. The therapist has a number of questions which he or she may ask in the context of other, more general questions.

Hearing and auditory skills

This section aims to identify the presence or absence of any hearing or auditory difficulties. If the client has difficulties with this, then his or her hearing requires in-depth assessment. The first items in this section assess the client's response to environmental sounds, such as the telephone or an ambulance. The items that follow assess the client's response to minimally contrastive sounds, with a bias towards the higher-frequency sound contrasts (sh/f, sk/sh, ch/sh), as these are the contrasts most often affected by intermittent hearing loss common among this population (Nolan et al., 1980). This section uses a series of black and white photographs and an audiotape of environmental sounds.

Vocabulary

The vocabulary section is a picture selection task which uses a series of black and white photographs, this time to determine specific receptive and, to a lesser extent, expressive vocabulary skills. The items in this section were selected from three word lists, two of which were based upon the oral vocabularies of adults with learning disabilities, and one upon an oral vocabulary list generated by adults without learning disabilities (Howes, 1966). They were tested in the three clinical trials described by van der Gaag (1988), and van der Gaag and Lawler (1990).

There are two lists of words, all of which belong to one of 12 semantic categories (after Crystal, 1982).These words are described as being either 'referential' (labels for an item) or 'attributive' (words which can be applied to a wide range of items, depending upon the context. For example, 'electric' can be used to refer to an iron, a kettle, a blanket or a television) (Swartz, 1977).

The expressive items in this section were selected on the basis of their functional use, as well as on whether or not they could be expressed using a sign or a gesture.

Comprehension of the functional use of everyday objects

This much shorter section examines the client's understanding of the functional use of everyday objects related to eating, washing, shopping and sewing.

Comprehension at sentence level (Sections 5 and 6)

Earlier sections looked at receptive and expressive skills at the single word level; these sections take on the assessment of comprehension at the sentence level. Section 5 uses object manipulation tasks, and Section 6 uses a picture selection task similar to the one used earlier to assess vocabulary. In Section 5, the verbal instructions are graded according to the number of 'information carrying words' (ICWs) (Masilover and Knowles, 1982) they contain. In Section 6, the client is assessed on his or her understanding of specific syntactic structures. These include intransitive, intensive, ditransitive, transitive/reversible and complex transitive verb structures, 'Wh-' questions, possessive pronouns and adjectives. Each structure is sampled once.

Communicative Functions

This section provides the therapist with a framework for observing the client's use of communication skills in a variety of everyday settings outside the one to one assessment context. It examines the same communicative functions as the carer: giving information, initiating a conversation, asking questions, describing events and feelings, telling jokes and stories (Chapman, 1972; Miller, 1978). It also outlines the basic 'rules' of conversation such as maintaining a topic, maintaining eye contact appropriately, the rules governing turn taking and physical proximity in a conversation. The therapist uses a rating scale to assess the client's abilities in this area.

Scoring

All of the subsections outlined above can be scored. The client's scores can then be looked at in relation to CASP's percentile rank chart.

Expressive skills

This section provides a summary of the client's expressive skills: his or her speech and/or gestures, symbol system, augmentative communication aid, intelligibility, fluency, volume pitch, rate and intonation. It is not scored, as it is a record of the therapist's ratings of these skills.

The CASP appendices

Concepts and social signs

'Concepts' is an extension of the second vocabulary list. It assesses the client's ability to understand attributes such as hot, cold, empty, sharp using black and white photographs. 'Social signs' examines the client's understanding of four 'social signs': 'Toilet', 'Danger', 'No Smoking' and 'Fire Exit'. The client is asked to select the appropriate sign.

Articulation

This provides the therapist with a more in-depth summary of the client's articulation skills. It allows recording of information of the client's phonetic and phonological systems (Ingram, 1976; Grunwell, 1985).

Imitation of gesture and oromuscular skills

There are two more appendices, one of which provides a summary of the client's ability to imitate gesture and the other a summary of his oromuscular skills.

Joint assessment

The final part of CASP is completed jointly by the carer and the speech and language therapist. It is essentially a summary of all the assessments made using Parts 1 and 2, plus any additional information from other assessments that have been made. It begins with a summary of the client's own perceptions of his communication skills. CASP recommends that, wherever possible, the client's own views of his or her communication should be sought. Does she or he think she or he has any difficulty in communicating with others? Does this make him or her afraid or shy or embarrassed about talking? The carer may well be the best person to discover these attitudes.

Strengths summary

The carer and therapist complete the strengths summary together. 'Strengths' have been divided into three areas: communication skills activities and resources.

1. Communication skills
   Hearing and auditory This includes a few sentences on the client's hearing and auditory skills. Comments on the client's attention skills is made here. Reference is made to Section 2 of the therapist's assessment in particular in completing this section.
   Understanding Therapist and carer summarise the information obtained from their assessments. To what extent does the client have understanding of single words? Does she or he appear to have better understanding of some words than others? To what extent is she or he able to follow verbal instructions? Reference is made to

Sections 1 and 3–6 of the therapist's assessment, and the first part of the carer's assessment.

Use of communication skills What is the client's primary means of communicating? How effectively can she or he get the message across? Is she or he intelligible? To familiars? To strangers? Can she or he initiate a conversation? Does she or he have a sense of humour? Does she or he show his or her feelings? How? When? Does she or he have an interest in communicating? Reference is made to the first part of the carer's assessment, and Section 7 of the therapist's assessment.

2. Activities in which the client is involved. Does she or he go regularly to any clubs, sports events? Does she or he have an interest in these? Does she or he join in or just attend? Does she or he have any particular responsibilities in the centre?
3. Resources. Information on the client's environment is summarised here. What education/skills training programmes is she or he involved in? What friendships are important to her/him? Who does she or he spend time with?

The communication environment rating scale

This scale is designed to 'help pin point how much communication the client is involved in on a day to day basis'. Some users of CASP have pointed out that this scale may seem intrusive to the carer, who is being asked to examine his or her own day to day interactions with the client. It may draw attention to the lack of interaction between client and carer. It is designed to do just that, to encourage critical and reflective thought on the part of all those who are in day to day contact with the client, including the therapist.

'Priorities for change'

This final section of the joint assessment is described as the most important part of the assessment process. 'Priorities for change' outlines the skills the client needs in order to communicate more effectively 'and therefore to live more independently' (p.68). The aim is to identify particular targets, and then to work out how those targets can be achieved. CASP suggests that the targets may fall into the following categories:

1. To carry out further assessments.
2. To identify a particular skill to be learnt.
3. To identify a particular aspect of the communication environment that needs to be altered in order to maximise opportunities for communicating.

Guidelines are provided on how to identify a particular skill, and stress that priority must be given to those that (a) the client is motivated to learn; (b) the keyworker is able to give attention to within the timetable of the centre; and (c) are relevant to the communication demands being made on the client (is there a gap between the client's communication skills and the demands that are made on him or her as a communicator? (Owings and Guyette, 1982).

Guidelines are also given on how to identify the 'criteria for success', in other words, how to determine when a particular targeted skill has been learnt, and is showing evidence of generalising to other contexts. This step by step planning before the implementation of the 'intervention' is seen as crucial to its success in bringing about change.

'Priorities for change' also records the details of who is to be involved in the teaching of which skills, and when the review of progress is to take place (Figure 4.1).

Personal Communication Plan (Hitchins and Spence, 1991)

The Personal Communication Plan (PCP) is a functional assessment and planning system which aims to involve 'as many relevant others as possible in looking at the communication of the focal person in the context of their everyday life and environment'. It has five sections, headed Background Information, Speech and Language Profile, Social Communication Skills, Environment and Shared Action Planning.

The PCP is divided up so that each section can be used independently. For example, the authors recommend that the first, third and fifth sections can be used in the assessment of social communication skills. Similarly, clients with little or no verbal communication, or who have challenging behaviours, can be assessed using the first, fourth and fifth sections. Each section contains a series of questions relevant to the topic, which therapist and carer work through together. Space is provided for comments, and identification of the action required in response to an identified need.

Theoretical basis

The Personal Communication Plan, in particular the section entitled 'Environment', is based upon O'Brien's five principles of normalisation (O'Brien and Tyne, 1981), These are used as a basis for describing the client's communication environment. Hitchins and Spence describe O'Brien's principles in their Introduction:

1. *Community Participation/Relationships*
This is the experience of being part of a growing network of personal rela-

STRENGTHS

This section should summarise the client's strengths.

SKILLS: Ask yourself how is she/he USING her/his communication skills?

Hearing and Auditory:
No significant difficulties. Assessments indicate adequate hearing and auditory skills. Attention good.

Understanding:
Very good understanding of common vocabulary and short sentences. Further assessments of size and prepositions required. Some difficulty recognising social signs.

Use of Communication Skills:
Initiates conversation easily, and will describe events and feelings without prompting. Communication is most effective when speech and signs are used together. Articulation is often difficult to understand. Eye contact, turn taking appropriate.

ACTIVITIES:

Social:
Goes to Tuesday club, makes regular visits to local shops and occasional visits to pub. Goes on holiday every year with other members.

Interests, Hobbies:
Very keen on swimming, and enjoys horse-riding. Goes to church regularly.

Responsibilities:
No responsibilities in SEC. In the hostel, she is responsible for her own money and medicines; for keeping her room tidy, washing clothes, etc.

RESOURCES:

Staff:
Good relationships with keyworker and with other staff in hostel, staff at SEC.

Family/Friends:
Good relationships with other members. No contact with family now.

Education Programmes:
Attends SEC daily. Social education, cookery, art.

PRIORITIES FOR CHANGE

SKILL	CRITERIA FOR SUCCESS	TEACHING METHOD	STAFF TO BE INVOLVED
To develop the use of speech and signs together to maximise functional communication.	*Use of speech and signs:* *a) prompted by keyworker.* *b) unprompted with keyworker, and staff in hostel first.*	*Keyworker and speech therapist to use speech and signs as example: combination of individual daily sessions and informal encouragement.*	*Keyworker. Staff in hostel. Other members. Speech therapist.*
Learn to locate in notebook and use as necessary her personal details e.g. address.	*Use of this with strangers:* *a) prompted.* *b) unprompted as necessary.*	*Keyworker to encourage her to use the information in her book.*	*Keyworker.*
Further assessment of size concepts, understanding of prepositions, and social signs.			*Speech therapist.*

Speech therapy involvement: *Weekly individual sessions. Fortnightly discussions with hostel staff.*

Review date: *31st October, 1987.*

Figure 4.1   CASP priorities for change

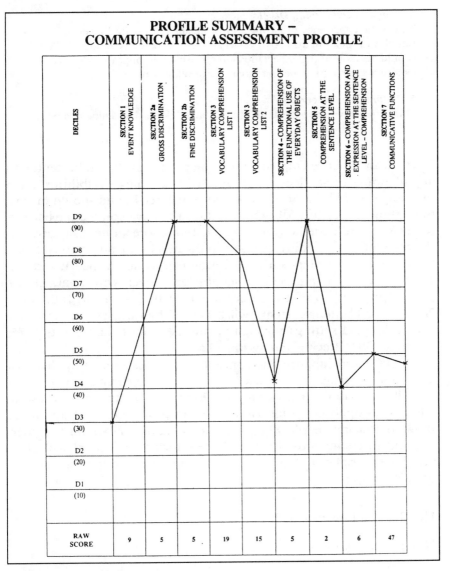

PROFILE SUMMARY – COMMUNICATION ASSESSMENT PROFILE

DECILES	SECTION 1 EVENT KNOWLEDGE	SECTION 2a GROSS DISCRIMINATION	SECTION 2b FINE DISCRIMINATION	SECTION 3 VOCABULARY COMPREHENSION LIST 1	SECTION 3 VOCABULARY COMPREHENSION LIST 2	SECTION 4 – COMPREHENSION OF THE FUNCTIONAL USE OF EVERYDAY OBJECTS	SECTION 5 COMPREHENSION AT THE SENTENCE LEVEL	SECTION 6 – COMPREHENSION AND EXPRESSION AT THE SENTENCE LEVEL – COMPREHENSION	SECTION 7 COMMUNICATIVE FUNCTIONS
D9 (90)									
D8 (80)									
D7 (70)									
D6 (60)									
D5 (50)									
D4 (40)									
D3 (30)									
D2 (20)									
D1 (10)									
RAW SCORE	9	5	5	19	15	5	2	6	47

Figure 4.1   *(contd)*

tionships which includes forming close friendships not only with other clients and service providers.

2. *Choice*
Choice is the experience of growing autonomy in both small and large matters. Personal choice defines and expresses individual identity, and people with learning disabilities should be consulted as individuals and should be part of any decision making process.

3. *Respect and Dignity*
This states that all people have the right to a valued place among a network of people and a valued role in the community.

4. *Competence/Personal Development*

This is the experience of having a growing ability to skillfully perform functional and meaningful activities whatever assistance is required. People should be allowed the expectations, responsibilities, opportunities, learning experiences and assistance necessary for development.

5. *Community Presence*

This is the experience of sharing the ordinary places that define community life.

Hitchins and Spence emphasise that the principles should be central to any planning of services for people with learning disabilities. Such planning should be centred upon individual needs, and should involve the setting of specific goals which will result in overcoming the barriers to living an ordinary life (King's Fund, 1980). The authors suggest that the assessment procedure can be coordinated by anyone who is directly involved in the client's life, but recommends that a speech and language therapist complete the section on speech and language. Its philosophy and format are very much in line with the Individual Programme Planning system, which is used by care staff in many day and residential settings throughout the UK (Houts and Scott, 1975; Dickens, 1983; Brechin and Swain, 1986).

The PCP also supports the concept of joint assessment by therapist and carer. It recognises the need to examine the client's environment as well as his functional communication skills. It supports the use of informal as opposed to formal assessment techniques, as 'experience shows that many people who have a learning disability tend to underperform in testing situations, and the information gained will often bear little relevance to how the focal person is communicating in everyday life' (p.4).

The five sections of the PCP

Background information

This provides a summary of the individual's cultural, social and physical environment. It includes questions about the individual's interests, hobbies, home circumstances, as well as details on any physical disabilities, relevant medical information on drug regimens etc.

Speech and language profile

This section is a checklist assessment of the individual's expressive and receptive skills. It gives an overview of the client's vocabulary, syntax, fluency volume, rate and intonation by asking the assessor to rate each in terms of either a strength or a need. For example, under the heading

'Vocabulary Size' the assessor is asked to consider how adequate the client's vocabulary size is for his or her everyday communication needs. She or he is then asked to rate this as either a strength (if no difficulties exist) or a need (if difficulties do exist), and to note any action that should be taken if a need has been identified.

Social communication skills

This section is a checklist assessment of the individual's non-verbal, verbal and assertiveness skills. Hitchins and Spence suggest that this is the 'key area' of communication for this population, because 'there is a high prevalence of skill deficit in social communication'. This section is therefore the most detailed section in the PCP. Each skill is rated on a five-point scale. The Non-verbal heading is concerned with assessing eye contact, facial expression, hand gestures, physical proximity, touch, fidgeting, posture and gait, personal appearance, volume, intonation, rate, clarity and fluency/hesitations. The Verbal heading includes listening skills, initiating skills, turn taking, asking questions, responding to questions plus other aspects of maintaining a conversation such as maintaining relevancy, and conversational repair and completion. Assertiveness skills include ratings on the the ability to express feelings and personal needs, to give opinions, to agree and to disagree, to make apologies and to make requests.

The information obtained in this section can be summarised on a pie chart similar in design to the one used in Gunzburg's Progress Assessment Charts (Gunzburg, 1963) (Figure 4.2). This provides a useful format for evaluating progress.

Environment

This section describes the environment in which the individual is communicating, using O'Brien's five principles of normalisation as a basis. For example, it asks about the client's relationships: 'With whom does the focal person spend most time? Are they people with learning disabilities or are they staff, family or other members of the community?' 'What would it take for the focal person to have more opportunities for contact with 'ordinary' members of the community?' 'How could we provide better support for the focal person in their present network of relationships?'

It asks questions about opportunities for making choices: 'How does the focal person make his choices known?' 'What would it take to increase the number of decisions the focal person makes?'

O'Brien's principle on mutual respect is reflected in questions such as 'Does the focal person have a valued role in their community across all aspects of their life, e.g. home, work and leisure?' 'Identify any

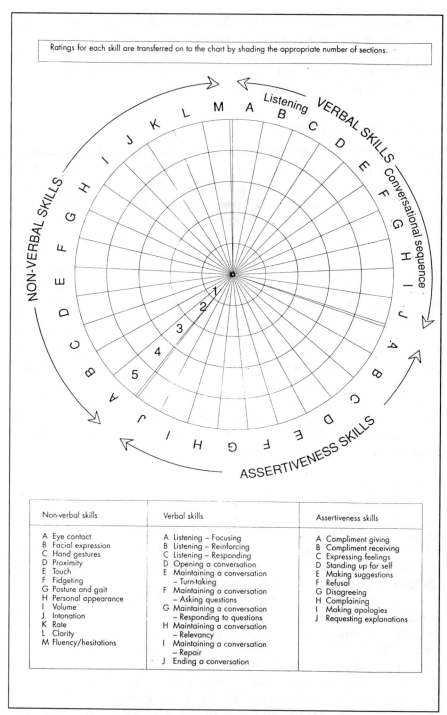

Ratings for each skill are transferred on to the chart by shading the appropriate number of sections.

Non-verbal skills	Verbal skills	Assertiveness skills
A Eye contact	A Listening – Focusing	A Compliment giving
B Facial expression	B Listening – Reinforcing	B Compliment receiving
C Hand gestures	C Listening – Responding	C Expressing feelings
D Proximity	D Opening a conversation	D Standing up for self
E Touch	E Maintaining a conversation	E Making suggestions
F Fidgeting	– Turn-taking	F Refusal
G Posture and gait	F Maintaining a conversation	G Disagreeing
H Personal appearance	– Asking questions	H Complaining
I Volume	G Maintaining a conversation	I Making apologies
J Intonation	– Responding to questions	J Requesting explanations
K Rate	H Maintaining a conversation	
L Clarity	– Relevancy	
M Fluency/hesitations	I Maintaining a conversation	
	– Repair	
	J Ending a conversation	

Figure 4.2 PCP social communication skills. (Reproduced from *Personal Communication Plan* by A. Hitchins and R. Spence (1991) with permission of NFER-Nelson)

barriers which prevent the focal person assuming a valued role in their community.'

Under 'Personal development': 'What are the barriers to the focal person developing skills?' (Consider personal issues such as health, motivation, communication, self-perception. Consider external barriers such as resources, support, staffing, stereotyped perceptions of disability.)

Under 'Community presence': 'What other facilities would the focal person benefit from using?'

A summary of this section is then completed before moving on to the final part of the PCP: shared action planning.

Shared action planning

This section provides a summary of all assessments of the individual's communicative needs, and outlines the steps required to meet those needs. For example, if the assessment has identified as a 'need': ' J. experiences little peer group interaction', the Action point would be: 'to increase J.'s experience of positive peer interaction'.

In their guidelines for this section, Hitchins and Spence stress the importance of reviewing progress at regular intervals. They recommend that this be carried out every 3–4 months. They also stress the importance of involving 'relevant others' in the shared action planning, and in setting very specific objectives or 'action', specifying how the action will be achieved, by whom, by what date etc. For example, if the action point is to 'Increase J.'s experience of positive interaction' then the steps to achieve this may be specified as:

Step 1   J. to join table tennis club at the centre.

Step 2   J. to be given responsibilities in his base group which will encourage interaction with his peers, e.g. to make tea/coffee in the mornings with Bill.

Each action point from each section of the assessment is numbered and cross-referenced where appropriate to other relevant action points. For example, the overlap between the items assessed under the Speech and Language section and the Social Communication section.

Encouraging a Natural and Better Life Experience:
ENABLE (Hurst Brown and Keens, 1990)

ENABLE is a systematic approach to the facilitation of the functional communication skills of people with a learning difficulty. It is essentially an intervention approach, incorporating an assessment schedule or 'profile', a 'programme' for intervention, and a 'resource' section, which gives step by step guidelines on different types of intervention. It is for use by speech and language therapists and carers and, like CASP and PCP, it stresses the importance of the carer's role in facilitating communication skills. ENABLE does not specify which ability level it is focusing on, presumably because it is designed for use with any adult with a learning disability.

ENABLE begins with certain assumptions. It assumes that every client, whatever the extent of his or her learning disability, has a definable set of communication skills and needs. It assumes that, with appropriate and regular facilitation, clients can 'tap their own personal potential and learn new skills'. It assumes that 'effective skill use in the majority of clients is markedly lower than potential skill use', in other words, that the majority of clients are under-using their communication skills. It assumes that, for many clients, the management of their communication must be viewed on a long-term basis. ENABLE also recognises the centrality of the carer and the 'communication environment'.

ENABLE is divided into four sections. The first is an introduction to the subject of 'communication', a training schedule for use with carers who are to be involved in the ENABLE approach. The remaining three sections, the Profile, Programme and Resource sections, are all subdivided into three levels: individual, group and location environment . The Profile section is a summary of assessments made on these three levels. Likewise, the Programme section deals with the identification of specific 'priority areas' (setting objectives for intervention), and the Resources section provides the ideas for 'facilitating' change at the individual, group and location environment levels.

Theoretical basis of ENABLE

ENABLE was developed by two speech and language therapists working with adults, who recognised the need for a functional approach to promoting communication skills. In their introduction, Hurst Brown and Keens (1990) describe their experience of the shortfall between supply and demand for speech therapy services in a large urban health district. They estimated that, as clinicians, they were providing a service to approximately 25% of the clients who were using day centres, when 'assessments revealed that 50% or more of these clients would significantly benefit from intervention of some kind'. This led them to re-examine their role as service providers, and to conclude that whereas detailed assessment of skills and needs should be carried out by a speech and language therapist, 'the resulting management on a long-term basis' should be undertaken by the carer. This, they argue, is because the carer has the strongest relationship with the client, and is therefore best able to adopt a consistent approach.

Implementing this rationale required the development of first, a framework for training carers, and second, a framework for intervention, incorporating goal planning and evaluation techniques that were meaningful to carers.

Description

The first stage in implementing the ENABLE approach is the recognition that its success depends to a large extent on the carers, who are already under considerable pressure to effect changes in other areas of their clients' lives. High staff turnover, low carer/client ratios, limited resources and facilities, limited training and staff support are identified as common experiences among staff in day and residential services. In recognising these, ENABLE provides a set of 'principles' which must be observed by senior staff (presumably service managers) and speech and language therapists, 'to ensure that the programme is neither impractical nor pressurising on carers'. The principles include statements about commitment to staff training on a regular basis, setting realistic and practical goals within the time and material resource allocation, a commitment to joint planning and regular support and liaison between carers and speech and language therapists.

ENABLE recommends reviewing the staff and speech and language therapists' attitudes to these 'principles' before embarking on any programme. This should lead to the drawing up of a 'contractual agreement' between therapist and staff, so that each is aware of the other's commitment, and presumably of the potential pitfalls that may arise once the programme has been implemented.

Training section

Having stated the principles underlying the success of the programme and achieved agreement between all those involved, ENABLE proceeds with a training schedule for carers on Communication. The topics covered by this include the nature of communication, the need for communication, augmentative systems, the skills associated with communication and the effect of the environment on communication.

Profile section

The authors describe the Profile section as a summary of the formal and informal assessments that have been carried out by the speech and language therapist in conjunction with the carer. They are not assessments in themselves, and should not be used as checklists. The three levels – individual, group and location environment – each contain separate headings, under which information is recorded. For example, the individual profile includes five headings: basic interactional skills, understanding, expression, the communication environment and the personal environment. Each heading contains a list of skills, all of which are given definitions in the manual. For example, eye contact is defined as 'the degree to which the client visually engages those with whom he is interacting'. The client's ability in all these areas is rated on a 0–5 scale by the therapist and carer, who go on to decide on a 'priority area' under the Programme section (Figure 4.3).

The same format applies to the group and location environment profiles. In the group profile, the therapist and carer are required to decide on their objectives for the group, and to compare all the group members' scores on the individual profile with each other. This information is collated on the summary of profiles of communication skills. The modal score for each skill is then calculated, which 'illustrates the level at which the majority of the group are functioning' in each skill area. This information is used in the selection of priority areas for the group.

In the location environment profile, the therapist and carers summarise information about the environment. ENABLE points out that this can be a threatening experience for carers. Therapists should be aware of this, and should allow the carers to decide on priority areas. The therapist's role is that of facilitator, not director.

The format for profiling the location environment is the same as for the individual and group profiles: a 0–5 point rating scale is provided for each aspect of the location environment. These are carefully defined in the manual (Figure 4.3). There follows a list of guidelines on choosing priority areas.

Programme section

The Programme section involves taking the priority areas from the three profiles and outlining the details of how these will be achieved. Ideally, a day centre or residential home should work on all three levels at one time, i.e. individual group and location environment objectives should all be pursued simultaneously.

Programmes are written by therapist and/or carer. ENABLE recommends working through the following stages in the writing of a programme, whether it be an individual, group or location environment programme:

1. The appointment of a key worker to coordinate the programme and keep all those involved updated.
2. The identification of all carers to be involved in the programme.
3. The determination of specific individual objectives, stating who will be responsible for what, how, when and where.
4. The determination of materials required to achieve the stated objectives.

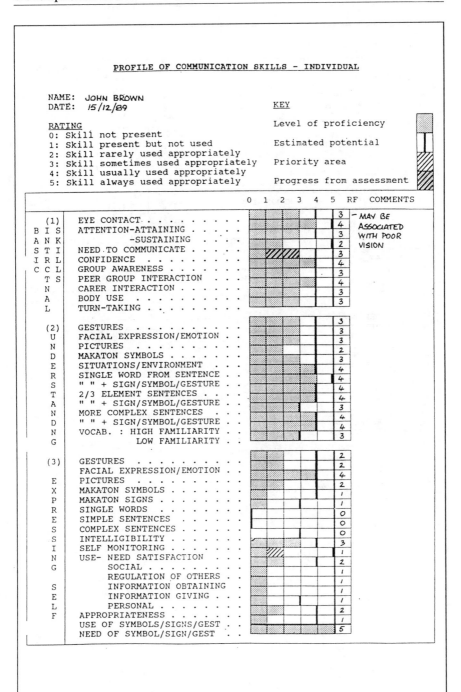

PROFILE OF COMMUNICATION SKILLS - INDIVIDUAL

NAME: JOHN BROWN
DATE: 15/12/89   KEY

RATING   Level of proficiency
0: Skill not present
1: Skill present but not used   Estimated potential
2: Skill rarely used appropriately
3: Skill sometimes used appropriately   Priority area
4: Skill usually used appropriately
5: Skill always used appropriately   Progress from assessment

		0 1 2 3 4 5	RF	COMMENTS
(1)	EYE CONTACT		3	– MAY BE
B I S	ATTENTION-ATTAINING		4	ASSOCIATED
A N K	-SUSTAINING		3	WITH POOR
S T I	NEED TO COMMUNICATE		2	VISION
I R L	CONFIDENCE		3	
C C L	GROUP AWARENESS		4	
T S	PEER GROUP INTERACTION		3	
N	CARER INTERACTION		4	
A	BODY USE		3	
L	TURN-TAKING		3	
(2)	GESTURES		3	
U	FACIAL EXPRESSION/EMOTION		3	
N	PICTURES		3	
D	MAKATON SYMBOLS		2	
E	SITUATIONS/ENVIRONMENT		3	
R	SINGLE WORD FROM SENTENCE		4	
S	" " + SIGN/SYMBOL/GESTURE		4	
T	2/3 ELEMENT SENTENCES		4	
A	" " + SIGN/SYMBOL/GESTURE		4	
N	MORE COMPLEX SENTENCES		3	
D	" " + SIGN/SYMBOL/GESTURE		4	
N	VOCAB. : HIGH FAMILIARITY		4	
G	LOW FAMILIARITY		3	
(3)	GESTURES		2	
	FACIAL EXPRESSION/EMOTION		2	
E	PICTURES		4	
X	MAKATON SYMBOLS		2	
P	MAKATON SIGNS		1	
R	SINGLE WORDS		1	
E	SIMPLE SENTENCES		0	
S	COMPLEX SENTENCES		0	
S	INTELLIGIBILITY		0	
I	SELF MONITORING		3	
N	USE- NEED SATISFACTION		1	
G	SOCIAL		2	
	REGULATION OF OTHERS		1	
S	INFORMATION OBTAINING		1	
E	INFORMATION GIVING		1	
L	PERSONAL		1	
F	APPROPRIATENESS		2	
	USE OF SYMBOLS/SIGNS/GEST		1	
	NEED OF SYMBOL/SIGN/GEST		5	

Figure 4.3   ENABLE Profile. (Reproduced with permission)

			0	1	2	3	4	5	COMMENTS
C O M M U N I C A T I O N	E N V I R O N M E N T	(4) SENTENCE LENGTH							
		VOCABULARY							
		AMOUNT OF LANGUAGE							
		RATE OF COMMUNICATION							
		USE OF INTONATION							
		USE OF MAKATON SIGN/SYMBOLS . . .							
		USE OF FACIAL EXPRESSION							
		USE OF GESTURE							
		USE OF CONTEXT							
		GAINING ATTENTION							
		GIVING ATTENTION							
		GIVING TIME FOR COMMUNICATION . .							
		ADEQUATE RESPONSE TIME							
		FACILITATING/CUEING ETC							
		OPPORTUNITIES FOR EXPANSION . . .							
		DEMAND FOR ACTIVE PARTICIPATION .							

(5) P E R S O N A L E N V I R O N M E N T			
	RELATIONSHIPS:	HOME	
		CENTRE	JANE IS A PARTICULAR FRIEND
		OTHER	
	PERSONAL LOSS		
	HEARING		
	VISION		PARTIALLY SIGHTED IN (L) EYE
	PHYSICAL		
	DRUGS		
	CHANGE:	HOME	JUST MOVED TO GROUP HOME
		CENTRE	
		OTHER	
	REALISTIC EXPECTATIONS:	HOME	
		CENTRE	
		OTHER	
	EXTREME LIKES/DISLIKES		DISLIKES LARGE GROUPS
	OTHER:		

Figure 4.3 *(contd)*

PROFILE OF LOCATION ENVIRONMENT

KEY

RATING   Factor level
0: Never appropriate
1: Rarely appropriate   Potential for change
2: Sometimes appropriate
3: Usually appropriate   Priority area
4: Always appropriate
                                Progress

ENVIRONMENTAL FACTORS	0	1	2	3	4

NOISE LEVEL/DISTRACTION
- External . . . .
- Large group-control . . . .
              -effect on indiv.
- Small group . . . .
- Leisure areas-control . . .
              -effect on indiv.

SEATING
- Position . . . .
- Type . . . .

ATMOSPHERE
- Large group . . . .
- Small group . . . .
- Leisure . . . .

GROUP DYNAMICS
- Group size . . . .
- Group composition . . . . .
- Level of abstraction . . . .

MOTIVATION FOR COMMUNICATION
- General environment . . . . .
- Group . . . .

AUGMENTATIVE SYSTEMS
- Use of signs . . . .
- Use of symbols . . . .

OPPORTUNITY FOR COMMUNICATION/
USE OF TIME . . . .

COMMENTS

90% OF STAFF HAD FULL MAKATON TRAINING,

WANT SUPPORT IN ACTUALLY PUTTING IT INTO

PRACTICE FROM THERAPIST.

Figure 4.3 *(contd)*

5. Choosing the first step of the 'goal plan'.This must be something that constitutes a step towards achieving the stated objective, and that the client can already do with some assistance.
6. Making reference to the Resource section, which gives guidelines on writing the goal plan for a specific skill.
7. Devising the individual goal plan using the relevant information in the Resource section, i.e. breaking the objective down into small, realistic steps).
8. Recording when each step is to be achieved, and when it is consolidated.

Resource section

The Resource section consists of step by step guidelines on how each skill summarised in the Profile section and outlined in the Programme section can be taught on an individual, group or location basis. The Individual Resource section gives a short explanation of the components of each skill, and then a specific example of how to 'programme' it. This is described in terms of 'general' and 'specific' facilitation techniques.

The Group Resource section follows the same format, although it does not contain any specific facilitation ideas. Instead of focusing on the teaching of individual skills, it is designed to 'facilitate the communication of clients within groups', either communication groups (discussion groups), or more generic groups, where members are there to learn other skills such as cooking, crafts etc.. There is no detailed goal planning here, as progress cannot be measured specifically in such settings. This section begins with general information on running groups, for example, the importance of having clear aims, of using rewards appropriately, of modifying one's own communication level to suit each client in the group.

The Location Resource section follows the same format as the Individual Resource section. Each location environment factor, such as noise levels in the centre, group dynamics, opportunities for communicating, use of time are all approached from a general and a specific point of view. For example, under the Motivation for communication heading, the general facilitation heading asks:

• Why is there limited motivation for communication?
• What effect is it having on the clients generally?
• What effect is it having on their communication?
• How much communication does occur?
• What precipitates it?
• How can we make communication a rewarding experience?
• How can we make communication at any level more necessary?

- How do our expectations of the clients match up to their actual capabilities?
- How can we adjust them?
- How important do we perceive communication to be among clients?
- How does expecting more communication from clients affect us in terms of time, energy, pressure etc.?
- What can we do in response to help us accommodate these?

The specific facilitation states that the objective must be, for example, to 'Establish one situation in which clients need to communicate (by reorganising mealtimes over the next two months)' by 'Ascertaining the way in which each client can show food preference at mealtimes (over the next week).'

INTECOM (Jones, 1990)

INTECOM is a package designed to integrate carers into assessing and developing the communication skills of people with learning disabilities. It is the first of its kind with a specific focus on developing carers' understanding and skills in relation to communication. INTECOM is not concerned with either the assessment or the teaching of specific skills. Its primary focus is on the individual's communication environment, specifically the scope and nature of relationships and the opportunities the individual has for communicating on a day to day basis. The package contains materials for group work with carers, a communication checklist for examining client/carer communication, and an 'opportunity planning' programme, which focuses the carer's attention on ways of increasing opportunities for communication.

The package is designed for 'interested carers' (which includes parents, friends, day care and residential staff, staff in further education colleges and special schools.) Originally, it was designed for use by speech and language therapists, but the author states that anyone who develops 'a thorough understanding of the INTECOM philosophy' and practice can introduce it to carers. Jones does, however, suggest that the best possible option is for the package to be used by a carer and a speech and language therapist together.

Theoretical basis

INTECOM is described by its author as an attempt to change the focus of speech therapy from an emphasis on the individual and his intrinsic communication skills to an emphasis on adapting aspects of the communication environment, thus enabling the individual's skills to be 'optimally used'.

Jones makes clear her opposition to the use of 'traditional' one to one speech therapy methods with this client group. She suggests that there is little evidence of the effectiveness of these techniques in bringing about changes in functional language use (Warren et al., 1980). She also states that

> Practitioners working in this field have recognised that many people with learning difficulties know much more than they communicate, often demonstrating their language skills in one situation but seemingly unable to use them across others. Indeed traditional structural approaches to language have severely underestimated the cognitive and social competencies which people with learning difficulties have. (MacDonald, 1985, (p.4)

Jones gives this as her rationale for shifting the focus of communication intervention away from a one to one setting and into an environmentally based approach. She acknowledges that speech and language therapists have already begun to implement this change by working much more closely with carers. However, she suggests that the wider issues surrounding work with this client group, such as the specific dynamics of how society at large devalues labelled groups of people 'has not been integrated into the literature, nor influenced the way speech and language therapists work'.

INTECOM is based upon three major tenets: that every behaviour, whatever its form, can communicate, and therefore every behaviour sends a message; that communication has 'cybernetic' attributes: it is essentially a 'feedback loop between two people who affect each other reciprocally'; and that self-fulfilling prophesy plays a vital role in determining the way that people communicate with each other. The expectations that one person has of another, and the way in which those expectations are perceived by the other, will have a profound effect on the nature and scope of the interaction itself (Jussim, 1986).

Jones suggests that this last principle has greatest relevance in 'substantiating the need to shift the focus of communication work to include carers' perceptions of people with learning difficulties'. She outlines the importance of people's expectations, and their subsequent influence on belief systems and behaviour. It is because people with learning disabilities experience difficulties in interacting throughout their lives that they are subject to negative perceptions of themselves, and to the negative expectations of others. INTECOM attempts to break down this common pattern by increasing the carer's understanding and insight, and by developing the client's ability to use his or her communication skills more fully.

Description

INTECOM has three sections: carer group work, opportunity planning and the communication checklist.

Carer group work

This section of the INTECOM package contains guidelines and materials for running five introductory training workshops on communication. The overall purpose of these workshops is to allow carers to explore their own perceptions of communication, and to look at how these influence the way they communicate with their clients. During these workshops the communication checklist is introduced to members of the group, and discussed in relation to specific clients. The manual provides a guide for the workshop facilitator, a structure for each workshop, and visual aids for use during each workshop. Jones stresses that the facilitator should take a non-directive approach to enable the participants to 'realise for themselves some of the themes that INTECOM advocates'. She recommends a maximum of 15 participants in any one group, and a minimum of nine. She also suggests that the most successful groups are mixed, with parents and professionals represented in equal numbers.

Opportunity planning

This section of INTECOM brings the issues and themes discussed by the carers into a direct relationship with the clients they work with. One of the outcomes of the workshops for most carers will be to identify those aspects of the environment that are not allowing the client to use his communication to the full. Opportunity planning provides a forum for discussing these in more detail, and devising ways of overcoming environmental constraints.

The communication environment is examined on three levels: relationships, daily routines and interactions:

1. *Relationships* Jones explains how people with learning disabilities often have 'an impoverished network of relationships' (Kings Fund, 1988). The first stage of opportunity planning is to explore this observation in relation to the carers and clients; the manual gives many practical suggestions of how this can be achieved. The objective is to allow carers to recognise the need to create more opportunities for clients to meet other people, and to make new friends. New relationships create new opportunities for communicating (Figure 4.4).
2. *Daily routines* This discussion point centres around identifying the positive and negative aspects of the client's daily routine. The section gives guidelines on how changes can be made on a day to day level. It also contains a daily schedule sheet for recording observations the carer makes. The first stage involves describing a typical day in the life of the client. Next the carer must ask: 'Which activities does the

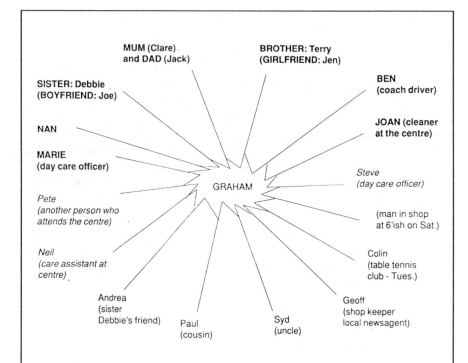

Key:
People Graham is in contact with daily
People Graham sees frequently but not daily
People Graham sees perhaps weekly

Seven people here are either family or paid staff.

In the second group are two paid staff and one close friend who shares Graham's interest in football and getting out of noisy break-times. Pete pushes Graham to the quiet room out around the outside of the Centre for fresh air.

In the third group, Syd and Paul are family but now and again they take Graham to watch the local football club. The man in the shop always seems to be around in the newsagents at 6.00 p.m. on Saturdays waiting like Graham and his Dad for the football results in the late edition of the local evening paper. This man always makes a point of directing conversation to Graham – this has always impressed Graham's Dad. Geoff the shop keeper is also a keen football supporter and once took Graham to an away match. On Tuesday evenings Graham goes to table tennis club at the local Sports Centre. Recently he has 'palled-up' with a young man called Colin, who at the end of the evening wheels Graham out to wait for his Dad to pick him up. Colin drives himself. Andrea sometimes goes to the club too.

IDEAS   1   Encourage links with Colin – could he drop Graham off after table tennis?
        2   Invite the man in the shop to go with Graham and Dad to the next home game.

Figure 4.4   Intecom opportunity planning. (Reproduced from *INTECOM* by Susan E. Jones (1990) with the permission of NFER-Nelson)

client choose and control?' 'With whom do they share this experience?' The next stage asks the carer to consider the concept of pre-empting in relation to the client's daily routine; this is where something occurs before the individual has had a chance to do otherwise. There are three types of pre-empting:

Environmental This is characterised by the arrangements of the physical environment which negate the need for language use, for example, when wanted materials and events are readily accessible, or when there is no opportunity to either change the pattern of what happens, or choose between items.

Non-verbal This is where other people anticipate a person's needs, desires and plans and fulfil them without requiring behaviour from the person.

Verbal This is where the person is communicating but other people around him or her inhibit communication by asking questions and providing prompts before the person can initiate.

Once examples of pre-empting have been identified, carers must ask themselves whether or not the pre-empting was necessary for the client. Alternatives are then sought and listed on the daily schedule. These alternatives provide the client with more opportunities to make choices and to have more control over his daily life, and reduce the amount of pre-emptive behaviour by carers (Figure 4.5).

3. *Interactions* The focus of this section is on examining the nature of the interactions between client and carers. The format is similar to the one used for examining daily routines. It involves looking at one or more typical interactions (either using videotapes or making real-life observations) between client and carer, and asking: 'When can the individual initiate communication?' 'When can the individual direct or change the course of the interaction?' Questions about pre-empting are then asked, and the carer decides whether or not the pre-empting is necessary in each instance. The final stage involves deciding on alternative strategies, listing how and when they may be implemented. An interactions profile is provided.

Sending clearer messages

The final part of opportunity planning provides a brief focus on the client's intrinsic communication skills. It provides the carer with a strategy for encouraging the client to 'send clearer messages'. This involves identifying a situation in which the client needs to communicate, and then observing which messages are required and used by people without communication difficulties (in that same situation).

The emphasis of sending clearer messages is not on changing the

Joan

Daily Schedule: Original list out

Date: 2 - 5 - 90

	Preempting	? needed
Bus picks her up from hostel at 9a.m.	E	No
Drops at centre 9.20 a.m.	E	No
Group Base room - collects cup of tea from tray	E	No
Group sit around and chat		
Makaton group / 'Conversation' group	N.V. * I decide	No
Breaktime. - all to main hall for coffee possibly snooker / records / quiet room		
Self-help group / Swimming (Tues)		
Lunchtime : set meal from canteen	E	? No
P.M. activities :		
(i) Women's group/cooking/current affairs (Rotate)	N.V. *	No
(ii) Keep Fit - Weights, Jogging, Netball, Football		
(iii) General chat/Reading/Knitting (few options)	E	No
(iv) Project work / Computers		
Bus arrives at Centre 4.15p.m. - back to hostel	E	Yes!?

Remember: try to be realistic – what actually happens in practice? It is useful to ask a colleague to check your account.

Published by The NFER-NELSON Publishing Company Ltd., Danville House, 2 Oxford Road East, Windsor, Berkshire, SL4 1DF, England.

Figure 4.5   Pre-empting

Joan

Daily Schedule: Revised list out

Alternatives	Possible message	Outcome

Make own way to centre
Other options to centre:
  ✱ Need to learn this
  COMMUNITY WORK EXPERIENCE
  LEISURE PURSUITS - LOCAL COURSES
    ↳ Pottery at comm. Centre

Lots! various

- state preferences
- indicate choices

To begin an summer pottery school at local centre - 2 days a week Aug & Sept.

Drink Making Facilities
Drink options

Ⓐ May
Build-in group planning for day
Expand options two 'experience' ✱

- state preferences
- discuss options
- argue within group

end June
Still developing
Lots of discussion
↓
beginning to get group decision &
Joan is active in this.

More choices in canteen - tackle staff !!

Make own lunch
  Ⓑ May
Go out for lunch - 'The Star' /
Eccelstall Prom Café

- specify preferences
- indicate decisions

explored options
keeping record
(took photos)

{ as in ✱

Indicate which alternatives are to be put into practice, and note down the date when this begins. Leave enough time for the changes to become established, between implementing the alternatives and recording the actual outcome. Date the outcome when recording.

NFER NELSON

Published by The NFER-NELSON Publishing Company Ltd., Darville House, 2 Oxford Road East, Windsor, Berkshire, SL4 1DF, England.

Figure 4.5   *(contd)*

client's communication so much as on refining existing alternative/augmentative communication strategies (facial expression, use of gesture, use of voice etc.). The manual provides ideas on how this can be achieved, first using video and role play, and then in real-life situations.

Communication checklist

The communication checklist is described by the author as a 'starting point' for carers in observing how the client is communicating (Section A) and what opportunities he has for 'sending messages' (Section B). The manual provides details of how this can best be achieved by the carer. Section A examines the client's level of motivation to communicate, his or her level of independence, primary mode of communication (speech, gestures etc.), level of expressive language, intelligibility and clarity. Section B records the carer's perception of how the client uses communication.

Comparison of the Four Assessments

Some of the more theoretical issues surrounding assessment have been discussed in detail in the preceding chapters. This section examines on a more practical level the strengths and weaknesses of each assessment.

In their critique of different methodologies used to assess the communication skills of adults, Dormandy and van der Gaag (1989) suggested that CASP did not go far enough in assessing the linguistic aspects of communication. The paper argued that assessments such as CASP should be used in conjunction with the therapist's own linguistic assessment 'using a number of phrases and sentences' which could 'elicit the desired linguistic forms'. The emphasis on functional assessment need not be at the expense of investigating specific linguistic structures. This argument had also been put forward by American writers, notably Calculator and Bedrosian (1988). It is interesting that PCP and INTECOM also pay little attention to this aspect of communication, and are more concerned with the so-called 'functional' aspects. The observations made at the beginning of this chapter about the nature of communication assessments, and in particular their linguistic components, have not really been addressed by any of the four assessments described above.

There are a number of commonalities in all four assessments which are worth noting. First, in contrast to IQ tests and standardised testing, the emphasis on working closely with carers is an essential part of all four assessment procedures. Each one states clearly that the carer is central to the assessment and intervention process. Each one creates a framework for involving carers. INTECOM and ENABLE include a training approach which allows carers to develop appropriate knowledge and skills; both are perceived by their authors more as training packages than as assessments. This focus on staff training as opposed to assessment is quite deliberate; INTECOM does this because it is not primarily concerned with the assessment or teaching of specific skills; ENABLE because it is essentially an intervention approach which includes an assessment or 'profile' section. Both approaches provide very useful structure and materials for training carers.

A second commonality is the emphasis on the 'communication environment' (Guyette, 1978). It almost seems taken for granted that this influence will be investigated, and yet the concept is a relatively new one in the context of communication assessment. CASP was the first assessment that included some kind of structured rating of the client's communication environment, but only provides a rating of the day and residential settings in terms of the opportunities for communicating with others, whereas INTECOM, the PCP and ENABLE provide more sophisticated frameworks for looking at the communication environment. INTECOM, for example, examines in depth the influence of the communication environment on three levels: the clients' relationships, their daily routines and the quality of their interactions.

The third commonality is that all four assessments place great emphasis on identifying specific communication needs, and on setting specific objectives with their clients. In other words, the assessment process and the intervention process are seen as parts of a whole. This approach has undoubtedly been influenced by the principles of goal planning, which are commonplace among other service providers working with people with learning disabilities (Houts and Scott, 1975; Dickens, 1983; Brechin and Swain, 1986). Each assessment uses a different label; for example, the PCP calls objective setting 'shared action planning', a term adopted from Brechin and Swain (1986). INTECOM discusses 'opportunity planning', CASP 'priorities for change' and ENABLE 'priority areas'. This trend is a positive one for communication assessments. It allows those involved to measure specific changes in whatever aspects of communication are the focus of intervention – the environment, the group or the individual. This is important not only because measurable goals are more likely to be achieved (Houts and Scott, 1975), but also because they serve as the outcome measures that public service managers are increasingly interested in (Normand, 1991). In other words, these measurable goals allow service providers to demonstrate their effectiveness in a particular task, an asset not to be underestimated in the current climate of increased accountability (Fratelli, 1986; Griffiths, 1988; DOH, 1989; Minifie, 1991).

Finally, all four assessments are designed for use with adults. They are age appropriate, and focus on the everyday aspects of language and communication in a variety of ways. They are all examples of what is commonly referred to as multidimensional, as opposed to one-dimensional assessments in that they all look at communication in different settings. Over and above these commonalities, each assessment has some additional features that the others do not have. For example, the PCP includes a focus on challenging behaviour, and on assessing individuals with little or no verbal communication skills. It is also based upon an existing framework for evaluating other areas of the client's life: the individual programme planning system. This makes it particularly 'user friendly' for carers familiar with this system. The INTECOM package contains a comprehensive, well organised training approach, with materials included. It provides an important focus on the influence of society's values and belief systems on the quality of services for people with learning disabilities. As Jones points out, this influence has 'not been integrated into the literature, nor influenced the way speech and language therapists work'(p.4). INTECOM also gives important guidelines on how to enhance the client's use of communication. ENABLE also highlights this by providing the most detailed, practical guidance on how to bring about changes in communication on three levels: individual, group and environment. CASP provides materials for assessing specific aspects of language, and a percentile rank chart for within-group comparisons.

To compare each assessment too closely can become counterproductive, as none of them sets out to achieve exactly the same objective in the same way. What is evident from this analysis and from the earlier descriptions of these procedures is that together they offer a particular perspective on communication which is long overdue in the study of communication difficulties (Halle, 1988). They reflect changes in outlook and practice which have also been taking place in the USA (Calculator and Bedrosian, 1988). They each have value as tools in assessment, and are a great improvement on the approaches that preceded them (see Table 4.1 for a comparison of the four methods).

In addition to the strengths and weaknesses of the individual profiles there are some properties which all linguistic and communication profiles share, some of which need to be questioned.

All profiles aim, explicitly or implicitly, at identifying the 'level' of communication a client exhibits. Yet we have no measures of competence, and therefore it is difficult to conceptualise how different 'levels' of communication should be characterised. The only thing we can be more or less certain of is whether it works or not. It is not easy to tease communication apart when it does work and state what made it work. It is, however, hoped that when it does not work it might be possible to identify what made it break down.

Another problem with all the existing profiles is that, despite claims to the contrary, none of them is in fact fully comprehensive. It is questionable whether comprehensiveness is a realistic goal. Crystal's (1982)

Table 4.1 Summary of the strengths and weaknesses of each assessment

Strengths	Weaknesses
CASP	

Strengths	Weaknesses
Focus on functional communication	Relies heavily on use of photographs
Intrinsic and extrinsic aspects of communication covered	Some aspects of communication skills are given little attention
Involves carers in assessment	Tries to cover too many aspects of communication
Strong theoretical basis	
Norm-referenced on UK adult population	Some sections rely on one-off response to a stimulus
Comprehensive clinical trials	Provides little practical help beyond assessment
Proven reliability and validity	
Age appropriate	
User friendly	
Carries no qualification restriction	
Makes specific statements about the aims and objectives of intervention, with review date and personnel specified	
Pre- and post-intervention measures included	

PCP

Strengths	Weaknesses
Focus on functional communication	Theoretical basis not explicit (besides reference to O'Brien's principles in relation to one section)
Focus on environmental aspects of communication	
Includes focus on challenging behaviour, and individuals who have little or no verbal communication skills	Reliability and validity of measure not tested
	Some questions too broad, especially re speech and language, articulation, vocabulary...how are these assessed? How are these questions answered? How detailed can the responses be without strategies for eliciting language?
Age appropriate	
Involves carers in assessment	
Easily linked in with IPP system (widely used in social services establishments)	
Flexible, discrete sections which can be used independently	
Makes specific statements about aims and action required, with review date and personnel specified	Introductory statements not substantiated by research, for example, what is the basis for statements on formal testing?
Could be used as a before and after measure, i.e. could chart client's progress on specific skills	
User friendly	
Carries no qualification restriction	
Useful as a basis for ongoing staff training	

Table 4.1 *(Contd)*

Strengths	Weaknesses

ENABLE

Strengths	Weaknesses
Focus on functional communication	Theoretical basis weak
Focus on environmental aspects of communication	No information on population tested on, for example, range of ability?
Age appropriate	No references to any other related work
Focus on intrinsic aspects	
Provides practical suggestions for intervention	Reliability and validity of measure not tested
Makes specific statements about the aims and action required, with review date and personnel specified	Overlooks phonology?
	Repetitive format in places
Pre- and post-intervention measures included	
User friendly	
Carries no qualification restriction	
Involves carers in the assessment and intervention	
Provides training for carers	

INTECOM

Strengths	Weaknesses
Focus on functional communication	Focus *ONLY* on the environmental aspects to the exclusion of the intrinsic aspects of communication
Focus on environmental aspects of communication	
Age appropriate	
Involves carers in assessment	Overstates the irrelevance of the one to one approach for adults with learning difficulties...where is the evidence?
Training package for carers structured, comprehensive, well organised, well laid out	
Pre- and post-intervention measures included	Reliability and validity data weak
Makes specific statements about action required	Assesses clients' functional communication at a somewhat superficial level – not a focus of the package
Carries no qualification restriction	

linguistic profiles are said to be comprehensive, which is only achieved by including the category 'Other'! Some of the other profiles do not even claim to be comprehensive. As Chapter 8 will show, it is not possible to provide for all eventualities in communication or list every single type of behaviour that might be relevant. Therefore, selection is necessary. But on what basis? Clearly the selection reflects the different authors' own personal focuses. Although this is perfectly acceptable for scientific enquiry in general, it may have the unfortunate consequence that it constrains the way we look at communication. It may attribute undue importance to some categories, and a diminished one to others. An even greater danger is that it may actually narrow down the scope of enquiry to just those parameters that the authors felt were important.

Lastly, whether or not the profiles are 'comprehensive' there is a tendency in all of them to look at all the listed components of communication, irrespective of their contribution to the overall picture. They do this in a piecemeal, component by component manner, with the result that it is impossible to form a coherent idea as to how a client in fact communicates. In order to arrive at a realistic picture of the communication abilities of a client it is essential to see the concerted functioning of the different components, and to observe what strategies a client is able to use to overcome a possible problem in one area by compensating for it in another. We hope to provide guidelines for the assessment of communication which avoids these pitfalls.

Part II
Current Issues in
Management

Chapter 5
Issues in Intervention

We now move into an exploration of management issues as they apply to work with adults with learning disabilities. One of the consistent expectations of any type of therapeutic initiative is change – change in the individual's communicative abilities, change in the way the individual communicates with family, friends and carers, change in the opportunities she or he has to use communication on a day to day basis. This chapter attempts to describe the elements that require attention if an individual is to communicate more effectively. It argues that the speech and language therapist needs to be aware of the wider social, psychological and environmental influences on an individual's ability to communicate, and must be ready to tackle change in any of these areas.

In Chapter 2 the importance of the characteristics of the participants involved in communication and the influence of context were discussed in relation to assessment. In this chapter, we look at the issues in intervention from a similar multidimensional perspective. First, from the viewpoint of the client in terms of his or her past experiences, personality, motivation and self esteem; secondly, from the viewpoint of the speech and language therapist and what she or he brings to the therapeutic relationship, and thirdly, the context or communication environment in which the client lives.

The Client

What are the common experiences of people with learning disabilities?

Much more is known about the experiences of people with learning disabilities than ever before, largely because they themselves are speaking out and telling their own stories. There is a great diversity in their lives and experiences (Atkinson and Williams, 1990). Trying to identify

the common experiences of people with learning disabilities is therefore something of a problem from the start. However, the purpose of
focusing on the commonalities that exist is to try and understand how
these experiences might influence an individual's communication skills.

All too often in the past the person with a learning disability has
been decentralised from the 'assessment' and 'intervention' process;
his life experiences have been made marginal to the 'linguistic analysis', or the 'clinical diagnosis' of the communication difficulty (Rowan,
1990). In the end, however, it is these experiences that shape the
expectations of the individual, his or her desire to interact with others,
to learn, to change and to communicate. It is also these that influence
the success or otherwise of any kind of therapy.

Much of the recent research on the subject of common life experiences comes from studies of people living in community settings,
either independently (Flynn, 1989) with their families, or in group settings (Edgerton and Bercovici, 1976; Reiter and Levi, 1980; Zetlin and
Turner, 1984). Much of it reveals a very negative core of common experiences, which of course vary from one individual to another. On a
financial level, it has been observed that people with learning disabilities frequently have low incomes and few personal possessions. They
have often experienced limited degrees of privacy, especially if they
have lived in large institutions. As children, they may well have become
aware that they are somehow different from other children, and have
experienced failure in one form or another (Dreeben, 1968; Hargreaves,
1978; Wilson and Evans, 1980; Barton and Tomlinson,1981).

Social isolation

One common experience of people with learning disabilities often
referred to is that of social isolation. Wiess (1975) commented that
'social isolation frequently occurs among individuals who are socially
stigmatised because of their handicaps'. Social isolation is often the
result of a limited range of the 'socialising experiences' to which non-
handicapped people are exposed, for example, visits to the pub, the
cinema, the bingo club, the sports centre or the theatre (Edgerton,
1975; Koegel, 1978). One of the consequences of this is that the individual is less familiar with many of the social skills that are used in
these settings and which actually make friendships materialise and
grow. Reiter and Levi's (1980) study of a group of people with learning
disabilities adjusting to life in a community setting concluded that one
of the characteristics of the group was a 'lack of social skills'.

Lack of continuity

A second common experience, linked with the experience of social isolation, is a lack of continuity in friendships and social support networks

(Richardson and Ritchie, 1989). Once people with learning disabilities move away from their families and into residential placements, they are often moved on into upgraded, larger or smaller facilities, without much consideration for the disruption this causes to the friendships they have established in each place. Flynn (1989) conducted interviews with 88 individuals with learning disabilities living in community settings, and found this to be the case for many of them. Companionship and friendship was perceived by these individuals as a valuable and important part of life, often interrupted by circumstances beyond their control. In some instances, these experiences can be linked with a sense of frustration at not being able to make friends easily or quickly. Kaufman (1984), in her study of people with mild learning disabilities living independently, quotes one woman who expressed it thus: 'I'm really normal inside and I don't know how to get that out to other people' (p.89). She felt very aware of being different and found it difficult to make friends as a result.

Richardson and Ritchie (1989) stress the need to recognise these and other barriers to the development of real friendships. For all human beings, friendships are an important context for self-expression. They are therefore very central to the use of communication. If people with learning disabilities often experience a lack of continuity in their relationships, then this will influence the ways in which they use their communication skills, and if it is as common an experience as the literature suggests, then it is an issue relevant to intervention.

Kaufman described the common friendship patterns of people with learning disabilities in terms of three categories:

1. Handicapped friends (friends with similar learning disabilities). These were friends in the day centre or social club, who shared the services and daily routines.
2. Reciprocal 'normal'/non-handicapped friends. These were neighbours, people encountered in shops, and other social settings.
3. Non-reciprocal friends. These were usually staff members in the day centre, social workers, other visiting professionals, employers, ministers etc.

The individuals with learning disabilities in her group who were rated with 'low sociability' had more non-reciprocal friends. Those with 'high sociability' ratings had the highest proportion of reciprocal friends. Flynn (1989) also observed that people with learning disabilities living in community settings made friends with paid staff more often than with 'reciprocal friends'. One example from her wealth of interviews illustrates this very well:

> Our friends come to see us...like the nurses who used to be at the hospital, they help us. They come and see us, Nurse Watkins and Sister Wilkinson come and see us. They used to work with us on B7, the babies' ward. And

Sister Bailey. Dave (social worker) comes down too, and Miss Curran, she used to be our Guide Leader. She used to have us in the Guides when we were small. On Wednesday and Sunday she still comes (p.82).

Flynn suggested that many of the individuals she interviewed showed a tendency to make 'friends' very quickly, and to assume that even the most transient visitor was a lifelong friend, or even a potential marriage partner, after one encounter. Many speech and language therapists will recall the experience of visiting a day centre for the first time, and being greeted as a close friend, often by more than one individual. One speech and language therapist recalled a visit to a centre that she had not worked in for over 6 months. As soon as she entered the building a client came up to to her and said 'Hello' and embraced her as though she had never been away. After a flood of questions, the client finally asked, 'What's your name, by the way?'

Rejection

The experience of rejection is also common to many people with learning disabilities (Miller and Gwynne,1972; Richardson et al., 1985). Miller and Gwynn point out that our physical appearance can often dictate how others react to us, and people with learning disabilities are no exception to this rule. Human beings often react differently to someone who looks or sounds different or unusual, or who has an obvious physical handicap. Even individual differences in weight can cause a negative reaction: people who are overweight can be ridiculed or experience rejection on this basis alone (Fox and Rotatori, 1982; Rotatori et al., 1983) The way in which this rejection is communicated to the individual in question will vary from overt avoidance to subtle changes in eye contact or physical proximity (Argyle, 1975). The reasons for this behaviour are complex, and are not the subject of this text. However, it is important to note that rejection is a common experience among people with learning disabilities, as it may well influence the use of communication.

Arguments in the past about individuals with disabilities not being sensitive to subtle but negative non-verbal signals are no longer part of the debate. The evidence against such views is strong, and the debate has now shifted to concerns about how these negative experiences actually affect peoples' lives and perceptions, particularly their perceptions of themselves (Bryan, 1986).

Victimisation

Victimisation of people with learning disabilities is another area of growing concern among practitioners and researchers alike. People with learning disabilities are no less sensitive to the negative attitudes of others, and many are now reporting experiences in which they have been ridiculed or victimised (Zetlin and Turner, 1984). Flynn (1989) gives this example of a couple who described what happened to them:

> I don't know why they just pick on us, nobody else here, just us. They've always done it, ever since we've lived here. It's nearly always different ones all the time...I've closed the curtains a few times and they've smashed the windows in. A pellet came through the window on New Year's Eve. It's a good job I moved out of the way quick or I'd have had a lump of glass in me back...Sometimes they take your washing off the line...I hate it. I don't mind the flat, it's just the area that I can't settle in. I'm dreading every night. I sit and watch telly and they're banging on the window...the police are here more times than they're not. I think they're fed up of seeing us the police...why do kids do it to some people and not to others? They've never bothered with that girl over the road or any of the others... (p.67).

Atkinson and Williams (1990) report similar experiences recalled by people with learning disabilities. One group of people composed a poem together, which they called *Tell them the Truth*

Tell them the Truth
There goes that mongol up the street
Getting on the looneybus
The schoolbairns call
Making funny faces at us
Calling us names
Headcase, spassy, wally
Nutter, Dylan, Twit!

There goes the dumbell into the nuthouse!
The schoolbairns are all daft themselves
They should see a psychiatrist
About their brains
It makes you mad, it boils your blood
Their wooden heads are full of nonsense.

They've got nothing else to do
Except make fun of us
We are human beings
And should be treated as equals
Treatment as adults
Tell them the truth.

Donald Lack, Robert Drysdale, Margaret Williamson, Derek Mustard, J.R. Grubb, Joan Cargill, Robert McMahon; St Clair Centre, Kirkcaldy (p.147)

The experience of victimisation was expressed more philosophically by Sean Rooney, quoted in Atkinson and Williams:

> When people take the mickey I feel very sad but not sad because people take the mickey out of me, sad because they are taking the mickey out of themselves.
>
> You want to know why I say that? Because if they've got something better to do, they wouldn't have taken the mickey out of handicapped people. But they don't have nothing to do all day but go round taking the mickey out of handicapped people (p.148).

Flynn's (1989) study supports Purkiss and Hodson's (1982) earlier work, which suggests that poor environmental conditions. Such as poor housing and few recreational facilities in the local community, are a major factor associated with episodes of victimisation like the ones described above.

Lack of choice

Many people with learning disabilities more often than not have had limited opportunities for making real choices in their lives (Guess, 1984). They will have become used to 'compliance' (Flynn, 1989) in small as well as large decision-making events. It was, Guess observed, as common for people not to be asked if they favoured resettlement in a group home as it was for them to be told that they were going on a visit to the local shops. They would simply be told what to do and when to do it. Changes in this area are still slow, but there are signs that service providers are much more aware of the importance of creating real choices for people. The influence of the self-advocacy movement has had much to do with this (Brechin and Swain, 1988).

Lack of structure

Florian's (1982) observations of a group of physically disabled people suggested that there was a link between a lack of structure in daily routines, and a general dissatisfaction with life. Other researchers have suggested an association between the development of challenging behaviours and a consistently low level of activity (Cullen et al., 1984). Graffam and Turner (1984) observed a group of adults in a sheltered workshop over a 2-year period, and concluded that boredom was the 'major expressed concern of the clients' (p.121). They also observed that clients' level of self-esteem and sense of social identity were directly related to the relative degrees of boredom they experienced over the 2 years. Lack of structure and consequent levels of boredom may, as with lack of choice, have become less commonplace in the lives of people with learning disabilities, but they may yet be the experience of many. In whatever context, not having enough to do will limit the subject matter of conversation.

'A broken self image'

Boredom, a lack of structure, limited choice in one's day to day life, victimisation, rejection, a lack of continuity in relationships and social isolation can lead to what Goffman (1963) called 'spoiled identity' and what Vanier (1982) later called 'a broken self image'. These experiences are, of course, not exclusive to people with learning disabilities. However, such individuals have often experienced these to a greater extent than the majority of people. One of the consequences may be low self-esteem (Atkinson and Williams, 1990). Zetlin and Turner (1984) comment thus:

> In a society which places high regard on mental ability and competence, it is difficult to imagine that an individual can be personally aware of his or her status as mentally deficient and yet remain immune to the associated stigma. It is more likely that individuals so labelled acquire identity standards which they apply to themselves (in spite of failing to conform to them), and which inevitably lead them to feel some ambivalence about themselves (p.118).

Zetlin and Turner are referring here to people with mild learning disabilities who, they observed, consistently denied that they were 'retarded', and whose ' reference group ', that is, those people with whom they consistently identified, were always people without learning disabilities (see also Edgerton and Sabagh, 1962)

How do these experiences relate to communication?

Several authors have stressed the importance of attending to the emotional components of communication, and the need to recognise the emotional and psychological needs of individuals who have difficulty communicating (Brumfitt, 1985; Miller, 1990). But do we make this a priority? Does our training encourage us to look beyond the 'clinical' analysis to the person and to their life experience? What the observations listed above highlight is that people with learning disabilities have often been subjected to negative experiences, which have shaped their lives and outlook and therefore their desire to interact with others. When we assess their ability to communicate, we often overlook this aspect of their lives, still less take these factors into account when planning intervention of any kind. This is not just true of speech and language therapists – it can be applied to all professionals. The fact that these experiences and their consequences are often overlooked can mean that unrealistic and inappropriate evaluations are made, and goals are set which do nothing to develop the individual's sense of well being or indeed sense of self. This kind of professional paternity often goes unrecognised.

There are many ways in which negative life experiences affect communication and how it is used. For example, one reaction is that a lack of trust of other individuals develops, and then manifests itself in a lack of interest in interaction other than the most basic communication of need. This can be the result of experiencing many short-term relationships in quick succession, or rejection by a loved one, or frequent personal insults. Another reaction to such experiences is to over compensate, to put a disproportionate amount of energy into trying to communicate with everyone. There are many variations in between these two extremes. Often an individual's way of communicating with different people will reflect this. Speech and language therapists may expect an individual to interact well with them because they are the expert on communication. From the client's point of view, they are also strangers, officials, visitors and, very often, testers. They demand conversation, words, answers. They may well be a reminder of some negative past experience.

Quite simply, this is an essential part of the person with the learning disability that 'professionals' often overlook or pay little attention to. Few speech and language therapists have drawn attention to this (Rowan, 1990). There is a danger that the focus of speech and language therapy involvement is not on the individual but on the process: the assessment, the goal planning, the review, the evaluation. The individual must remain central; the development of his or her sense of self and right to self-determination are paramount (Brechin and Swain, 1988). Atkinson and Williams (1990) provide this summary:

> A sense of identity is not easily achieved. People with learning difficulties are faced with obstacles at every turn. Their stories witness their battle, often life-long, to overcome these obstacles and find a sense of self. The battle is both against outside forces (often well meaning parents and carers) which deny adulthood, and internal learned prohibitions (particularly the internalised barrier to parenthood). The struggle finds expression in the search for, and celebration of, freedom and independence (p.217).

The Therapist

There has to date been relatively limited attention given to intervention from the speech and language therapist's point of view, and how this may affect success in therapy. Recent research in related fields such as aphasia therapy have begun to look at this aspect in more detail (Byng, 1990). There are, of course, a number of clinicians who place great emphasis on the psychodynamic aspects of therapy, and whose way of working with clients will reflect this (Brumfitt and Clarke, 1983; Miller, 1990). Our concern here is to look at intervention from the therapist's viewpoint, to examine some of the issues that affect the way he or she works, and how the professional client relationship affects therapy, before examining some of the different models of service delivery in Chapters 6 and 7.

The so-called traditional methods of intervention – one to one, once weekly speech and language therapy – are not by and large favoured by speech and language therapists specialising in work with adults with learning disabilities, according to Jones (1990) and Hitchins and Spence (1991) They suggest that these methods are not effective with adults. Perhaps a more accurate analysis would be that they have no proven effectiveness, and certainly they have little social validity among many clinicians.

The uncertainty about what does and does not work has contributed to the change in how speech and language therapists working with this group view themselves and their contribution. New methods are being tried, new ideas experimented with, new frameworks are emerging all the time (Jones et al., 1992) Where does this leave the therapist? How does she or he feel about the changing role? What kind of conceptual framework can she or he use, which encompasses all these (sometimes radical) changes, while at the same time giving a sense of purpose and achievement in what she or he does?

One way of creating a conceptual framework is to view speech and language therapists as individuals who have many different personas, who after all belong to what has been called a 'polymath profession' (van der Gaag and Davies, 1992a). They do not belong to the medical model of intervention and yet they have medical knowledge, much of it very specialised. Equally, they do not belong to the education model of intervention, and yet they use teaching techniques. They have knowledge of the psychological influences on human behaviour, particularly in relation to human communication. They are skilled in a variety of assessment and therapeutic techniques, and are able to offer diagnostic information when required. In some sense, the speech and language therapist takes on these different 'personas' of teacher or carer, and at different times they may be more one than the other. Some of these 'personas' are explored below.

The speech and language therapist as teacher

In some ways, newly qualified speech and language therapists probably feel most confident in the role of teacher. They have learnt to use specific teaching techniques, have the skills necessary to make decisions about what activities or tasks might be appropriate, and know how to introduce these activities to the client. However, they may not be aware of the complexities of these skills, nor indeed that they are teaching skills at all. Saunders and Caves (1988) conducted an in-depth study of speech and language therapists' skills, and found that they were using a very broad range of skills in their day to day clinical work, without necessarily being aware that they were using them. Skills such as reinforcing, modelling, shaping, cueing, mirroring, which many experienced speech and language therapists almost take for granted as part of their therapeutic repertoire, are in fact highly complex teaching skills.

It was noted by van der Gaag and Davies (1993) that therapists are often not aware that they have teaching skills: when they are asked to list the skills they use, they find it difficult to name these as 'skills' without prompting. It may be that, as more and more therapists are asked to train carers, they will find it essential to externalise these skills so that they can be shared more successfully with others. This may also lead therapists to recognise the importance of their role as 'teachers', not just of clients but of carers as well.

The speech and language therapist as carer

This role is probably the least well defined, and the most commonly exercised. Speech and language therapists are frequently viewed as having a 'supportive' role, both with clients and carers, and by clients and carers. They provide direct and indirect counselling, and their role is often to affirm and encourage (Pickering, 1987; Anderson, 1988; Egan, 1990). Miller (1990) has highlighted this role in her discussion of the speech and language therapist attending to the emotional and psychological needs of clients. It is very difficult, Miller argues, to separate communication from affect. The consequences of a communication difficulty will be linked inextricably with the emotional and psychological balances within the individual. It will also have emotional and psychological consequences for the people who interact with that individual. There can be little doubt that the speech and language therapist does have responsibility to attend to these aspects of the communication difficulty, and that her role as 'carer' in the sense of providing such support is often a vital one.

The speech and language therapist as supervisor

This role develops out of spending time training other members of the team in the use of specific teaching and therapeutic techniques. It is a role which has received very little attention in the literature, considering its importance to the success of so many skills sharing exercises (Pletts, 1981; Pickering, 1987; Anderson, 1988; Green, 1992). There is evidence that without ongoing monitoring and appraisal, staff who have received in-service training will not sustain new learning in the long term (Cullen, 1988). What they may need is continuing (but not continual) feedback sessions and discussions about intervention, sometimes formally, and at other times informally. For this, the speech and language therapist must develop supervisory skills. These skills, according to Rose (1991) are very similar to counselling skills. They include establishing and maintaining confidentiality, trust, empathy and understanding. They also include the ability to be non-judgemental, challenging and supporting. Well developed listening skills, problem-solving skills and self-awareness are also part of supervisory skills.

The speech and language therapist as supervisee

Supervision should not only be seen in the context of supervising carers. Increasingly, therapists are recognising the importance of attending to their own supervisory needs. The growth of therapists' support networks is beginning to receive more attention. Green (1991, 1992) and Rose (1991) describe the development of a cross-district supervision network in Riverside Health Authority which aims to provide mutual support for all therapists. Rose (1991) points out that other professional groups already have well established support systems, for example, psychiatry, psychotherapy, social work and counsellors of various sorts. Speech and language therapy has been slow to recognise its own needs in this area. Green (1992) gives guidelines for how such support groups might operate. For example, she recommends fortnightly meetings of no less than six therapists. They should ideally meet for an hour and a half. Topics might include case discussions, problems with colleagues or personal problems affecting work. A facilitator might be appointed to lead the group. If possible this person should be someone who is not a speech and language therapist. Green and her colleagues are presently setting up a mutual support network between occupational therapists and speech and language therapists, so that members of each profession can act as the others' facilitators.

The speech and language therapist as team member

There is yet another role that speech and language therapists need to acknowledge as important – their role as a member of a team. This may be a difficult role for a therapist who has previously worked alone in a community clinic to adopt. It may be the reason why some therapists feel that they achieve limited success in their work with adults with learning disabilities: they are reluctant to integrate themselves fully into working as part of a team of people who have very different skills and backgrounds. This is not always the fault of the individual therapist, however. It may well be that other members of the team are reluctant to accept the speech and language therapist's input, however humbly or assertively it has been offered. However, there must be a team approach for intervention to be successful. The therapist needs to spend time building relationships with other members of the team, and establishing a role within it before she or he can hope to achieve any lasting effects with clients.

The speech and language therapist as a 'resource'

It is often the case that the speech and language therapist takes on the role of a resource worker, someone who acts as an 'agent' in acquiring a particular service for a client. This is particularly true when clients require a communication aid, a hearing assessment or a hearing aid, as these are resources which play an important part in securing successful communication. This is less of an incidental role than one might think. One recent survey of hearing skills in a population of day centre users found that all the clients with Downs' syndrome and 60% of all other clients wearing hearing aids had external auditory meatus problems (excessive wax, infection etc.) (Pinney and Ferris Taylor, 1989). This was only discovered because the speech and language therapists working in the centre conducted their own survey of hearing skills; they argued that hearing assessment was a necessary precursor to any communication intervention. In the absence of an audiometrician, they screened the total population themselves, and then referred on those clients whom they felt required a more in-depth hearing assessment. This may be considered an unusual role for a speech and language therapist to take on, but given limited resources it may be an essential prerequisite to delivering an effective and an efficient service.

The problem of limited resources

The problems surrounding limited speech and language therapy resources will be dealt with in more detail later on, but it is worth introducing the topic in this context because limited resources extend beyond speech and language therapy: they affect all the public services to people with learning disabilities. This in turn affects the role of the speech and language therapist. There has been much discussion as to the overlap between various members of the team, and doubtless there will be yet more now that the Community Care Act has come into force and the social services assume an even greater responsibility for the delivery of services. What is important for the speech and language therapist in terms of deciding on a role, or planning a particular strategy, is that she or he and whoever else may be involved with the client has identified the most qualified person available to take on that particular role or task. In other words, that it is not an ad hoc decision, but is based on a proper analysis of the *resources available from all the agencies concerned.* It is only by focusing on such issues that we can begin to identify when and where additional resources need to be allocated.

If we use this framework for conceptualising the work of the speech and language therapist with adults with learning disabilities, we may find it easier to accept and develop the multidimensional non-linear approach. The kind of role confusion experienced by many therapists may, in fact, be due to a reluctance to embrace all these roles, rather than trying hard to fit into one or the other. Why should there be one role, or one direction for speech and language therapy intervention with adults with learning disabilities? Why not many? Perhaps the most crucial question for each individual therapist, and particularly for those new to working with adults with learning disabilities, is not what is the role of the speech and language therapist, but which role do I recognise/feel most comfortable with? Which role do I feel I need most help in developing? What role do the people I am working with have for me? Is there a mismatch there? These are the sorts of questions which may need to be addressed, along with questions about what techniques are most appropriate for which client. Establishing one's own persona as a therapist, recognising one's own needs and preferences in a professional context, is equally important to successful intervention (Green, 1992).

Some questions which may be helpful to this process of self-reflection are suggested below. It may be helpful to go through some of them in a small group context.

Which of the following roles do I feel most comfortable in?

- Teaching?
- Caring, supportive, counselling?
- Supervisory?
- Being part of a team?
- Working alone?
- Directing others?
- Being directed by others?
- Planning?
- Practical side of therapy?
- Researching?
- Working with other therapists or without them?

Can you rank order them?

- Which of the above do you feel least comfortable with?
- What kind of situations do I find most difficult to deal with in the day centre? Residential setting?
- Can I identify the reasons why? What do I feel when I'm about to arrive at the centre?
- How much time do I spend at the moment in the role(s) that I enjoy? What could I do to increase this time? Could I get help in developing my training skills/my supervisory role with carers?

The locus of control in the therapeutic relationship

Finally, therapists need to remind themselves of just how powerful their role is. In any professional/client relationship of this kind, the main source of control is the professional. However, the extent of that control will depend very much on the theoretical orientation of the professional as well as on personal characteristics and experience (Rogers, 1951; Egan, 1990; Jacobs, 1990; van der Gaag and Davies, 1992b). Whatever their orientation, therapists have a substantial amount of power, which frequently promotes dependency on the part of the client. This outcome can conflict with the overall aim of therapy, which must be to facilitate independence and to let the client take responsibility for his or her own life. This is a relatively new concept in the field of learning disabilities, which is being debated in relation to many topics: employment, leisure, economics, sexuality, to mention only a few. The issue of power in the context of therapeutic relationships is hopefully not a new concept to speech and language therapists. They have been made aware of this in their training in the dynamics of the therapeutic relationship. The challenge for the speech and language therapist is to recognise that the client therapist relationship in this context faces the same issues of power, control and dependency as for any other group, but more so because of the contexts in which people with learning disabilities live and the spoiled identity which they often share. A lack of self worth can lead to a sense of powerlessness. It is therefore all the more crucial that the therapist is aware of the dynamics involved and guards against promoting this kind of dependency (Langer, 1983; Brechin and Swain, 1988; Wootton, 1992). Brechin and Swain (1988), in their discussion of professional/client relationships, point out that, in general, the greater the learning disability the more controlling the professional relationship is. This has implications for the outcome of intervention as well. The focus on achieving independence becomes virtually impossible if the client is never given opportunities to develop control over his or her own environment. To put this into the context of developing communication skills, there needs to be an emphasis on providing the client with opportunities for initiating, directing and controlling the immediate environment, by whatever means – verbal or non-verbal.

The Communication Environment

Having looked at the experiences of people with learning disabilities and the role of the therapist, we now focus on the environments in which adults with learning disabilities might live. Much of the literature has concentrated upon the effects of particular physical environments, such as hospital versus community-based environments (Lyle, 1960; Zigler, 1961; King et al., 1971). As fewer and fewer people are now living in hospital settings, the focus of research has shifted towards closer analysis of particular features of the environment, such as the quality of the interactions between staff and clients (Cullen et al., 1984), the opportunities that clients have to exercise choice in their day to day living, (Evans et al., 1987) and the relationships they develop (Flynn, 1989).

In what way has this influenced speech and language therapists?

This focus on different aspects of the environment has influenced the way in which speech and language therapists look at an individual's communication skills quite considerably. Speech and language therapists working with people with learning disabilities now refer routinely to the client's 'communication environment', as if it had always been a focus of attention. It is in fact a relatively recent concept. Guyette (1978) first used the term to refer to those aspects of the environment which would influence an individual's ability to communicate, for example, the opportunities to use communication skills on a day to day basis, and the demands that were made on him or her to communicate. Turner (1982) and others from the Socio Behavioural Group at the University of California talk about environments having 'personalities' which need to be explored and defined in the same way that human personalities might be. Recently developed communication assessment and intervention packages have begun to take account of this, and include formal strategies for examining the communication environment (van der Gaag, 1988; Hurst Brown and Keens, 1990; Jones, 1990; Hitchins and Spence, 1991).

This is, however, a relatively recent change in the way we look at communication. It may be useful, therefore, to consider how and why this change has come about. Egan (1984) provides some helpful insights. He suggested that there are historical reasons why the cultural and context-based influences upon the individual have traditionally been either ignored or overlooked by the 'helping' professions. He provides this illustration:

> A person walking beside a river sees someone drowning. This person jumps in, pulls the victim out, and begins artificial respiration. Then another drowning person calls for help. The rescuer jumps into the water again and pulls the second victim out. This process repeats itself several times until finally, much to the amazement of the bystanders who have gathered to watch this drama, the rescuer, even though the screams of yet another victim can be clearly heard from the river, gets up from administering artificial respiration and begins to walk upstream. One of the bystanders calls out: 'Where are you going? Can't you hear the cries of the latest victim?' The rescuer replies: 'You take care of him. I'm going upstream to find out who's pushing all these people in and see whether I can stop it'.

Egan's point is that this 'helper' changes his strategy once he realises that there must be something causing these human casualties – he seeks out the 'malfunction' in the system, rather than continuing to try and intervene on an individual basis. In much the same way, speech and language therapists working with people with learning disabilities are seeking changes in the so-called 'communication environment', which in turn will lead to changes in the opportunities which the individual has to use his or her communication skills on a day to day basis.

Egan goes on to ask why the helping professions have for so long adopted the 'downstream' approach, focusing almost entirely upon the individual. He offers two explanations: first, he suggests that there is a dependence on the 'medical model', which defines the individual's 'problems' in terms of types of 'illness' which require 'treatment'. As discussed elsewhere in this text, this is a largely inappropriate model for people who are not by definition ill and do not require medication or hospitalisation any more regularly than the rest of the population.

Egan's second explanation relates more widely to Western society's focus upon the individual rather than the sociocultural system. This remains a peculiarly Western focus, in stark contrast to the predominantly community-based focus of Asian and African cultures, for example. In the West, attention is directed towards individual thoughts, feelings, values and behaviours. Both of these preoccupations have driven the helping professions into a person-oriented approach, often to the exclusion of environmental influences on communication.

In essence, Egan's thesis is that human development is a function of the interaction between people and the 'human systems', or environments, in which they are involved. He defines 'human systems' as the groups to which individuals belong: family, school or college, place of work, pub, club, community, country or government system. Egan goes on to say that, in order for the remedial professions to maximise the quality of the interaction between the individual and the system, they need to have a working knowledge of the way systems work, as well as knowledge of the developmental processes that shape human behaviour. The 'helper' must also have the kind of 'life skills' – interpersonal skills, self-management skills – that facilitate these skills in others. Egan claims that 'helpers' of one kind or another, often do not have this knowledge or these skills. It may be that speech and language therapists have an in-depth knowledge of developmental processes – physical, emotional, psychological, cognitive and linguistic – but they have not to date had as much awareness of this knowledge of people in systems which Egan describes: an awareness of the way in which human systems work, and how they affect human development.

What kind of framework or structure can we use for looking at human systems, or environments? Egan's 'people in systems' model suggests that there are four 'levels': personal systems, the interaction of different personal systems, organisations and institutions, and the wider cultural level.

Using the people in systems model

Personal systems

This refers to the most immediate settings, such as family, college, place of work, pub, club, church etc. The quality of interactions in these settings will have a profound influence upon the individual's development. The literature on family therapy bears this out (Goldenberg and Goldenberg, 1980). Andrews (1974) gives a very clear illustration of the family as a system (Figure 5.1).

> In a family of four...there exist six dyadic reciprocal relationship possibili-
> ties. These tie each member of the family to every other member directly
> and indirectly...One might construct a physical model of this diagram by
> using paper clips to represent each family member, and connecting rubber
> bands to represent the relationship vectors in the diagram.... Plucking any of
> the rubber bands will reverberate the entire model. Similarly, any action or
> reaction pattern between any two family members will resonate throughout
> the entire family.... The 'family resonance' phenomenon is the perpetuating
> mechanism of characteristic behaviour within a family. Reinforcement of
> certain kinds of behaviour is not unilateral or even bilateral but multilateral
> (p.8).

Those familiar with a group home setting in which people with learning disabilities live will see the parallel here. The links between the 'paper clips' and the' rubber bands' in the group home may not be as permanent as they are in the family setting, but the principle of resonance is the same.

The network of personal systems

This level reflects the interactions between the different personal systems that any one individual is involved in, and how the interactions within one such system influence interactions in another. For example,

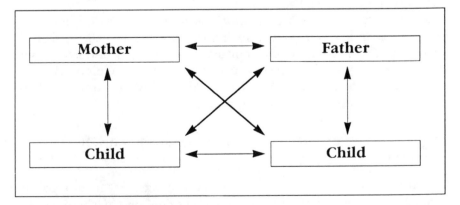

Figure 5.1 The family as a system

an individual who has an argument with a friend in the day centre may go home feeling angry or upset, and this will affect his interactions with the people he goes home to that evening.

The organisations or institutions of society

These systems affect our lives both directly and indirectly. For example, if the travel budget for the day centre is cut, then the people attending will no longer have the same opportunities to use local amenities. Local policies regarding what people attending day centres can and cannot do varies quite considerably: in one local authority for example, people with learning disabilities can choose to go on holiday anywhere at home or abroad. Another local authority dictates that they are only permitted to organise holidays within certain geographical boundaries, because the authorities say that 'the norm' for people living in the locality is 'local' holidays – local people cannot afford to go abroad, so why should people with disabilities have that choice?

Culture and its systematic effects

Egan refers to 'cultural blueprints' which shape peoples' lives – in effect, ways of behaving within a particular culture. This is particularly relevant to people who may be moving from a hospital to a community setting: their experience of living in an institution will be very different from the experience of living in a community. The cultural blueprint will affect almost every aspect of their lives, from what they eat to what they do with their time. One man who had recently moved from a hospital to a community setting complained when he was given a plate of spaghetti bolognese that it wasn't real Heinz spaghetti, like the spaghetti he had eaten in hospital: 'It's not real spaghetti we get here – it's all long and disgusting, not like Heinz. I like Heinz spaghetti best.' To many of us, the reverse would have been true – spaghetti out of a tin would not be the real version!

What the 'people in systems' approach provides us with is a framework for expanding our view of the individual with a learning disability into the wider societal or sociocultural context. It is important that speech and language therapists widen their frame of reference in this way in order to maximise the changes that allow the individual to become a more effective communicator.

What aspects of the communication environment must be examined?

In many ways, existing communication assessments do not go far enough in examining the wider human systems or environments to which the individual belongs (van der Gaag, 1988; Hurst Brown and Keens, 1990; Hitchins and Spence, 1991). Their focus is on the first and second levels outlined in the people in systems model – the network of personal systems and how they interact with one another. What we are suggesting is that the speech and language therapist needs to be aware of the organisations and cultures to which individuals belong, and to take these into account when planning opportunities for change. However abstract these concepts may seem, they exert an enormous influence on people's everyday lives.

Looking at the organisation and the culture

Perhaps the most practical way of looking at these systems is to examine the policy, structure and resources in the setting receiving (or about to receive) a speech and language therapy service.

Policy

Policy issues in relation to services for people with learning disabilities include such things as the 'operational policy' of the day or residential setting, its 'mission statement', its general service delivery policies. Is it geared towards providing opportunities for integration into community life? Does it recognise that clients have diverse needs? Does it recognise the importance of identifying those needs and then providing a means of meeting them? Does it express a commitment to allowing clients to make decisions about their own lives? Is the centre committed to seeking local employment for clients? Is it viewed as separate from, or part of, the local community?

Structure

Looking at the structure means making an assessment of the day to day running of the day centre or residential setting. The different roles and responsibilities of the staff and clients need to be clarified. Who organises what in the centre? What are the main activities? Are activities largely centre-based or community-based? How are roles and responsibilities divided up in the home setting? Does the centre use the Individual Programme Planning (IPP) system? Is there a balance between work and leisure activities?

Resources

What resources are available to clients in the centre or residential setting? What opportunities do they have to use local community resources like the leisure centre, shops, library, college, adult education courses, arts centre, theatre, cinema or clubs? What are the links with these community resources? Are they considered important? What links exist with local groups? Are attempts made to offer the centre to local arts and other adult education groups for their own evening meetings? What are relationships with neighbours like? What links exist between day centre and home environments?

Staff

The most important resource in any day or residential setting is the staff group. The speech and language therapist would therefore do well to spend time with the staff, both individually and by attending staff meetings on a regular basis. Very often, speech and language therapists will spend time attending staff meetings initially, but will not continue to do so because they feel they are wasting valuable time. Yet regular contact between people working within an organisation is seen as one of the most crucial elements to its success (Handy, 1975; Peters and Waterman, 1982). Initially, the speech and language therapist needs to discover who are the 'leaders' and who are the 'followers' in the staff group. Which members of staff are interested in communication as a subject? Which staff member recognises and points out that a particular client is being prevented from developing independent living skills because his communication skills are limited? What is the management's commitment to allowing staff to develop their particular skills and interests? What is the management's view of training? What training has been provided in the past?

These are the sorts of questions which the speech and language therapist should have in mind when establishing his or her role within a particular location. They serve as 'scene-setting' devices initially, but in the end they shape the nature and the extent of speech and language therapy intervention for all the clients.

Chapter 6
Issues in Service Delivery: I

The total environment, or culture, in which individuals with learning disabilities live can have a major influence on both the method and the success of speech and language intervention. This chapter looks at the environmental influences from two quite different perspectives. First, in terms of the current philosophies which may shape the individual's environment, and second in terms of the various settings in which services are typically provided.

Philosophies

Normalisation

The principle of 'normalisation' was first put forward by Bank-Mikkelsen (1969), Director of the Danish Mental Retardation Service. He defined it as 'letting the mentally retarded obtain an existence as close to the normal as possible'. In 1959 this principle became part of Danish law relating to services to people with learning disabilities (Nirje, 1969).

It was not until 1972 that Wolfensberger published an extensive document on the subject in English. His name has been associated with the term ever since, and he has been instrumental in providing both theoretical and practical exposition of the principle. Many other researchers and service providers have contributed to the literature on normalisation (Nirje, 1969; Grunewald, 1971; O'Brien and Tyne, 1981; Welsh Office, 1983; Brechin and Swain, 1986). As a result, it has become the most widely discussed principle behind the provision of services to people with learning disabilities in the UK and the USA. More recently, it has been renamed 'social role valorisation' or SRV (Wolfensberger, 1983).

Wolfensberger (1980) described SRV as a meta theory, in that it is a simple statement whose corollaries influence the way in which services are delivered on both a structural and a systemic level. It is, in fact, a principle that can be applied to any service delivery system, but it is perhaps most powerful when applied to services to people who are 'devalued' by society.

There are many definitions of the principle: Wolfensberger (1980) himself gives three, which he says operate on different levels, but have the same meaning:

1. The use of culturally valued means, in order to enable people to live culturally valued lives.
2. The use of culturally normative means to offer people life conditions that are at least as good as that of average citizens and, as much as possible, to enhance or support their behaviour, appearances, experiences, status and reputation.
3. The utilisation of means which are as culturally normative as possible, in order to establish, enable and support behaviours, appearances, experiences and expectations which are as culturally normative as possible.

Social roles

The principle of normalisation, or social role valorisation as it is now known, relies upon several concepts, which relate to society's precepts on peoples' social roles. We are all aware, to differing degrees perhaps, that we come to every social encounter with certain precepts which will determine to some extent our response to that encounter. When it comes to encounters with 'devalued' people, these precepts can have a particularly strong influence (West and Ansberry, 1968).

The first of these relates to what Wolfensberger (1980) calls 'role circularity', or role definition. If the role definition imposed on a person is a negative one, then that person is perceived as 'deviant'. Negative role definitions can arise from a person's physical characteristics, for example, physical features, poor posture, old age, or from his or her past or present behaviour, social skills, cultural habits, beliefs, or from his or her background, for example, nationality or descent. One powerful example of a negative role definition was a report in *Community Living* of four families in Hertfordshire who bought a £160 000 house in their street to prevent it from being bought for use by six individuals with learning disabilities. They were convinced that the value of their own homes would drop by £30 000 if these individuals became their neighbours. The resident who led the campaign said that he had to 'protect' the street (Community Living, 1990).

The second concept relates to what Wolfensberger calls 'role images'. Once the person has been given a negative role definition, there is a strong likelihood that he or she will receive a subsequent role image, for example, 'the subhuman', 'the object of pity' or 'ridicule', the 'eternal child', the 'sick person' etc. These role images are highly correlated with various types of service; for example, the 'sick person' will require a 'medical service' provided by 'doctors, nurses and therapists'. The 'eternal child' will require 'protection' provided by a 'parent'. Negative images are more likely to be attached to devalued people than positive images. For example, elderly people have a negative role image in Western societies, because old age is not associated with vitality and good health, which are highly valued in the West. One consequence of this is that advertising uses very few images of elderly people to sell consumer products.

Wolfensberger argues that the medical model of service is one of the most powerful in use in Western society. The devalued person is 'sick' or 'diseased', medical personnel make 'diagnoses', and prescribe 'treatment' in 'clinics' or 'hospitals'. No-one would suggest that there is no place for the use of medical terminology. Apart from anything else, medical specialisation and advancement could not continue without them. What Wolfensberger and his colleagues challenge is the negative role images that are associated with their use and over-use, and the devaluing effect of this upon the person who receives the service.

If service providers are to enable people with learning disabilities to lead culturally valued lives through the use of culturally valued means, then, Wolfensberger argues, they must be aware of these concepts, and must consciously work towards enabling the people they serve to have access to all the social, leisure, work and community activities that are enjoyed by people who are 'culturally valued'.

Misinterpretations of normalisation

Brechin and Swain (1988), in their excellent analysis of the nature of professional–client relationships in relation to normalisation and the self-advocacy movement, suggest that there are two common misinterpretations of the normalisation principle. The first is the notion that normalisation is about 'making people normal' (Sinha, 1986). Normalisation was never intended as a basis for developing behavioural and objective-based intervention, with an emphasis on changing people's behaviour regardless of what they might want. There is a danger that techniques such as goal planning and individual programme planning, which do not consider first the needs and opinions of the individual, promote this kind of professional paternalism.

The second misinterpretation occurs when normalisation becomes a way of 'packaging' an individual's life, of being prescriptive, of becoming focused on providing ordinary housing, ordinary transport, ordinary leisure activities because these things will make him or her more 'acceptable' to society. Brechin and Swain describe this as some kind of 'marketing' strategy, which loses sight of individuals and their needs. In the end, these kinds of change lead to confusion and disorientation rather than enabling the individual to have more control over his or her own life.

The essence of normalisation is that it recognises the individual's right to self-determination and personal autonomy. The challenge for professionals is determining how best they can facilitate that process.

The advocacy movement

The advocacy movement developed in parallel with the development of normalisation. Whereas the normalisation movement grew out of academic and professionally held ideas, the advocacy movement had quite different roots. It began in the USA in the late 1960s, when 'self help' pressure groups organised by people with disabilities began campaigning on civil rights issues. Many of the early campaigners were veterans from the war in Vietnam. The issues the movement brought to the attention of politicians and the public included equal employment opportunities, equal access to leisure facilities, public transport, housing, insurance and credit services (Braddock and Fujiurah, 1991). People with disabilities did not receive the same employment opportunities as other people, they argued. They did not have easy access to cinemas, cafes, restaurants, theatres and sports facilities. They had difficulties obtaining ordinary housing and necessary mortgage and insurance services. Decisions about where they lived, who they lived with, who they formed friendships and intimate relationships with, how they spent their time, what clothes they wore, were all decisions taken largely without their involvement. In effect, people with disabilities began 'speaking for themselves', highlighting their need for better benefit systems, legislation and real opportunities to live 'ordinary lives', to make their own decisions, to increase the range of choices available to them. As a result of this campaigning in the USA, antidiscrimination legislation for disabled people was gradually introduced. The most recent of these, the Americans with Disabilities Act (1990), is by far the most radical commitment to creating a society free of discrimination against disabled people. In all likelihood, the advocacy movement and its supporters in the UK will achieve a similar legal precedent in time.

The underlying principle of the advocacy movement was, from the outset, to create opportunities for self-determination (Brechin and Swain, 1988). In many respects, this initiative was no different from initiatives by the feminist movement and the black civil rights movement. In common with other pressure groups working for oppressed minorities, the advocacy movement has not always been taken seriously by 'the professionals' (Dowson, 1991). Comments like 'Our service users aren't ready for self advocacy' and 'We are planning to set up a self-advocacy group for the more able adults' undermine the whole principle of self advocacy. Professionals were rightly accused of being patronising when they attempted to initiate self-advocacy groups. This is because the principle is not to make decisions for people but to empower them, to give them the means and the opportunity to achieve things for themselves.

There is much evidence that people with disabilities are achieving this aim. 'People First', the largest network of self-advocacy groups run by people with learning disabilities in the UK, began in 1972. It now has a regional structure, allowing individuals and groups to take local action against discrimination, and to be proactive in dispelling misconceptions and fears among their neighbours, to lobby for more appropriate local and national policy and legislation. For example, the Calderdale People First group was involved in campaigning against a private entrepreneur who wanted to open a 40-bedded home for people with learning disabilities in the locality. The People First group made it clear that this type of accommodation did not constitute 'ordinary' housing; it was simply establishing another 'mini institution'. The home was never opened (Values into Action, 1991).

Some advocacy groups invite non-disabled people to act as 'advocates' for individuals who have difficulty communicating and have chosen to have an advocate to help them to make their views known. Elsewhere, peer advocacy networks are being implemented, in which a group of people with learning disabilities organise an advocacy service for their peers (Brandon, 1991). The common element in all these initiatives is that people with learning disabilities are deciding what they want, and service providers are responding, rather than the other way around.

The sociopolitical nature of the movement is another feature shared with other minority rights groups. This can also help to create mistrust or even hostility between its members and members of professional groups, who may see themselves as apolitical. However, without this political focus, the advocacy movement would have made little progress in establishing better opportunities and more equal relationships for its members. Issues such as housing rights, rights to better employment opportunities, rights to parenthood, have all been placed on the political agenda by people with learning disabilities through advocacy organisations. It is interesting that the professionals who are least supportive of local advocacy initiatives rarely see the movement in the wider context of consumer sovereignty, which has become such an important part of British society and thinking in recent years (Pfeffer and Coote, 1991) Without consumer pressure, environmental issues, such as wasteful packaging or lead pollution, would not have received such widespread attention from manufacturers and politicians alike. Indeed, the current proliferation of Citizens' Charters (HMSO,1991a,b) has emerged from a recognition that 'the consumer is king', that the consumer has rights and opinions that should be listened to and respected by policy makers (Pirie, 1991). These concepts are not new: they are simply more commonplace now. They underpin the potential power and influence of all pressure groups and organisations, of which the advocacy movement is one.

The extent to which speech and language therapists become involved with local advocacy initiatives will depend entirely upon the individual therapist. Some have chosen to become involved with the movement by providing members with training in literacy and assertiveness skills, or by acting as advocates for those who have difficulty communicating verbally, or by encouraging greater understanding of learning disabilities among the local community. One speech and language therapist described her involvement in helping to secure a job in a supermarket for a man who used Makaton to communicate. She provided Makaton training for the supermarket staff so that they could communicate with her client. This man would never have started work had he not had the support and enthusiasm of an advocacy group and the willingness of the therapist to be involved.

At the extreme end of the advocacy continuum are those who can find no role for the professional, and who are not prepared to support any cooperation between professionals and people with learning disabilities because the very existence of professionals helps to perpetuate society's view of the person with a learning disability as 'helpless', 'powerless' and therefore 'oppressed'. Chapter 5 touched on some of the dangers inherent in any therapeutic relationship. There are undoubtedly power struggles and dependency relationships being played out between speech and language therapists and people with learning disabilities, just as there are for other related professionals (Brechin and Swain, 1988). The advocacy movement, with its emphasis on the rights of people with disabilities, has done much to raise awareness of the dangers of this type of oppression. It has made a significant contribution to the changes in services for people with learning disabilities. (For more practical information on self advocacy, the reader is referred to Palmer and Dawson, 1992.)

Have normalisation and the advocacy movement influenced the delivery of speech and language therapy services to people with learning disabilities?

The introductory chapter of this book discussed the influence of paradigm shifts on the practice of speech and language therapy. There are certainly shifts in the pattern of service delivery which mirror the more widespread changes in services brought about by the influence of normalisation and the advocacy movement. Two illustrations of this are described below.

Terminology

The vast majority of speech and language therapists and their assistants in the UK are employed by the National Health Service. Those who choose to specialise in work with people with learning disabilities have undergone the same initial training as their counterparts in general hospitals and community health centres, where the medical model is applied. Speech and language therapists in the hospitals and health centres talk about 'patients' and 'dyspraxics', 'dysarthrics' who attend 'treatment sessions', and who are 'admitted' and 'discharged' from 'therapy' in much the same way as patients are 'admitted' and 'discharged' from surgical wards or radiotherapy treatment. In contrast, speech and language therapists who work with people with learning disabilities are much less likely to find a use for these medical terms. They point out that people with learning disabilities are not 'sick' and do not require 'treatment' or 'rehabilitation'. Rather, they are individuals who require specialist help in order to enhance the quality of their lives. There is a very different emphasis in the terminology used here, and it is not difficult to make a link between this change in emphasis and the normalisation principle.

Direct to indirect therapy

As has been noted elsewhere (Scott et al., 1987) there has been a shift towards working more closely with carers, and focusing upon other aspects of the communicative process beside the client's intrinsic abilities.This shift can also be linked to the normalisation principle. Wolfensberger noted that the process of devaluing can be reversed in two ways: by minimising the differences or stigma of deviancy that activate the perceiver's devaluation (intrinsic influence), and by changing the perceptions or values of the perceiver (extrinsic influence). It is no coincidence that the emphasis in speech and language therapy intervention has been more and more on the second of these. A recent study of the skills and competence of speech and language therapists working with people with learning disabilities (Davies and van der Gaag, 1992b,c; van der Gaag and Davies, 1992b,c;) made several observations that reflect the shift from direct to indirect therapy. It was observed that:

1. Medical knowledge and the application of medical techniques and expertise formed a relatively small percentage of the total knowledge and skill base required of the speech and language therapist working with people with learning disabilities. Knowledge of educational and psychological techniques took up a much larger proportion of expertise than medical knowledge (see Appendices I–XIII).

2. Decision-making processes concerned with assessment and intervention planning were more likely to be based on environmental (or extrinsic) factors, such as opportunities for communication, or organisational support for intervention measures, than upon factors intrinsic to the person's communication skills, for example the existing severity or degree of difficulty.

Types of Service Provision

This section has been written for the therapist who has little or no experience of working with adults with learning disabilities, and who is unfamiliar with the types of service available. Over the last 10 years, the shift away from institutional care has resulted in the development of a wide variety of community resources for people who previously lived in large mental handicap hospitals in both the UK (DHSS, 1971, 1981; NDT, 1976), and the USA. This shift has had enormous consequences for both service users and service providers. The move away from institutional care combined with the impact of normalisation and the advocacy movement has resulted in adults having more opportunity to have control over their own lives, making their own choices about how they spend their time, where they will live and who they want to live with. For the service providers, be they health or social services or privately run establishments, the shift has required major changes in the manner in which services are delivered at all levels: location, content, aims and objectives.

There is little doubt that this change of policy towards adults with learning disabilities has resulted in vast improvements in the quality of life that can be achieved. However, as with all services, there are geographical variations in the pattern and the quality of community-based services. The examples given below represent a small cross-section of services in the UK.

Day services

Day centres for adults with learning disabilities are generally funded and managed by the social services departments. There are fewer examples of day services run by health authorities, and equally few run by independent charities or private concerns. Those run by health authorities tend to provide services for people with high dependency needs, whereas social services establishments tend to provide for adults with varying levels of need living within a certain catchment area.

Day centres are called by a variety of names, from the more traditional 'Adult Training Centre' or ATC, to Social Education Centre, Resource Centre, or Day Centre. Others prefer to be called by a name such as 'The Avenue' Centre, which does not identify them as readily as a centre for people with learning disabilities. Labelling depends largely upon the attitudes of service providers and service users.

Typically, day centres provide a service for between 40 and 150 individuals. Below are some specific examples.

The Adult Training Centre

This description of a 'typical' day service for adults with learning disabilities is taken from Williamson's (1991) ethnographic study of a day centre.

The ATC is situated on an industrial estate on the edge of the town. It was built in 1970. It looks very much like the other industrial units around it: originally the building was fitted with a loading bay and a conveyor belt which allowed the centre to cater for the large amount of contract work undertaken. This would range from putting buttons into plastic bags to assembling car components. The centre prides itself on its work for local industry. In addition to the rooms set aside for contract work, there are rooms used for other purposes, for example, an art room, a woodwork room, a kitchen area, a garden/allotment area, three 'education' rooms, a kitchen and dining room and various office rooms. There are separate toilet and cloakroom facilities for staff and trainees. In addition to the main site, there is a 'skills unit' on the other side of the town, which consists of an ordinary house used for training purposes.

The individuals who attend the ATC are known as 'trainees'. The majority come to the centre each day by coach or taxi. Very few use public transport. At the moment, 120 trainees attend the centre, which is staffed by 14 full-time and two part-time 'instructors' (staff). The skills mix of the staff is varied, but with a high level of academic qualifications: five have higher degrees, one is a registered nurse and seven are undertaking further study (for example, City and Guilds qualifications, Certificate in Social Services).

Each trainee has an annual review during which goals are set and a timetable of activities is decided upon. This review will be attended by the trainee, his or her parents and/or carer, his or her keyworker, a social worker, and the centre manager or deputy manager. The trainee will be allocated a keyworker from among the staff group as soon as he or she arrives at the centre, and is then a member of a particular keyworker group in the centre.

The daily routine in the centre is very structured. Trainees arrive by coach or taxi between 9.30 and 10 a.m. They will go to their keyworker group for the first 45 minutes of the day, and will then begin the day's activities according to their individual timetables. Virtually all activities are based in the centre. A small number of trainees who are moving into more independent living accommodation will visit the 'skills unit' (a flat on the other side of town) on a regular basis for further training in independent living skills such as household and cooking tasks, use of public transport and local amenities etc. However, for the majority of trainees, a typical timetable might look like this:

	Monday	Tuesday	Wednesday	Thursday	Friday
Morning	Woodwork	Cooking	Contract work	Art	Education
Afternoon	Self care	Garden	Contract work	Social skills	Disco

The day is broken up by a coffee break in the morning and a tea break in the afternoon. Lunch will be served in the dining room. The day ends at 3.30 p.m. when coaches and taxis arrive to take the trainees home.

Wye Centre

The Wye Centre is described by its Manager as a 'resource for day services to adults with learning difficulties'. It was opened in 1989, a new building catering for 55 clients and 14 members of staff. It is situated in a residential area of a small town, 10 minutes walk away from busy high-street shops. The building itself centres around a small courtyard, decorated by a large wooden sculpture. There are several large rooms, one of which is used as a dining area, another as a craft room. The smaller rooms in the building include a pottery room, a photography dark room, a kitchen area and a TV room. There are a number of offices and a cloakroom. Outside there is a garden area, which has been taken over by the sculpture project. Funded by the Gulbenkian Foundation, professional sculptors and people from the centre are working together to create new sculptures in the grounds.

At any time during the day, more than half the clients are out of the centre. The range of activities open to them is extensive: there are sporting activities such as horse-riding, swimming, athletics, football, netball, keep fit, table games, basketball and walking. There are educational opportunities in the local further education college: courses in literacy, cooking, crafts, dressmaking, using computers. There are work experience opportunities ongoing in a nursery garden, an old persons' home, a supermarket, a bakery, a hotel and a farm.

Activities inside the centre include home economics (cookery, shopping, home care, budgeting), personal care (hygiene, hairdressing), crafts (dressmaking, tapestry, needlework, candlemaking, rugmaking), art (using many different media), aromatherapy, music, woodwork and gardening. In addition, topics covered under social education and social skills development include literacy and numeracy, social sight vocabulary, community awareness, Makaton and other forms of communication, self advocacy, the development of relationships (personal and sexual), families and friendships, and coping with bereavement and loss.

In addition to these ongoing activities, the Wye operates a cooperative which produces crafts such as dried flowers, silk cards and jewellery. These are made on the premises and sold to shops, offices and factories. The cooperative is now looking for new premises away from the centre.

The building itself is available to the general public for rent in the evenings and at weekends. It is used by the local Further Education college as a venue for short courses in pottery, photography, calligraphy, soft furnishing and yoga among other things. It is also used for plays and play rehearsals, dances and community meetings.

Every 3 months clients have an opportunity to decide which activities they would like to be involved in as part of their individual day service programme. The IDSP, much like the individual programme planning system, provides a record of the client's aims for the next year, what he or she would like to achieve, etc. These aims are expressed as specific goals; for example,

AIM: I would like to work.
GOAL: To get work experience at the local supermarket once a
        week.

Wherever possible, timetables are organised according to the client's stated aims. A typical 3 month timetable for an individual client might look like this:

	Monday	Tuesday	Wednesday	Thursday	Friday
Morning	Coop Work	Social skills	Working in supermarket	FE college (art)	Cookery/ riding
Afternoon	Social skills	Self-care course	All day	FE college (art)	Aroma- therapy

Each staff member is a 'linkworker' to five clients. As linkworker, he or she is responsible for ensuring that clients' timetables are helping them to meet certain learning objectives outlined in their individual day service programme. In addition, each staff member is part of a team responsible to clients living in a particular geographical area. Part of the team's responsibility is to plan travel and activity budgets for their client group. The management give the staff considerable autonomy in this respect.

Wherever possible, clients make their own way to the centre each day. Although the centre has a minibus, transport is usually by car or bus or on foot. Clients use the local shops and cafes as part of their regular routine. They use the libraries, leisure centre, pubs, parks, cinemas. They are offered real choices for ordinary life experiences.

Increasingly, day services for people with learning disabilities are not focused in one building but in the community. In contrast to the ATC described by Williamson, the Wye Centre activities are based in the community as well as in the centre itself. This means that local amenities such as shops, libraries, leisure centres and community centres are the settings for developing personal interests and exercising choice. The individuals who use the centre are encouraged to use local facilities in the same way that any other member of society does. In normalisation terms, they are encouraged to enjoy the same ordinary life experiences as other people.

More radical approaches to service provision in the community

A community-based service

One health authority in London established a more radical approach to working with adults in the community. Its service consisted of 12 full-time staff who worked with 12 individuals living in two staffed houses, rising to 15 full-time staff and 15 individuals living in four staffed houses. There was no day centre facility besides office accommodation for the staff and two large rooms in the office building, which were used for group activities and meetings. All activities besides those which took place in these rooms were community-based, making extensive use of educational and leisure facilities in the district. This is an example of a service which successfully put the principles of normalisation into practice. It provided support in the community, which allowed the individuals concerned to live 'an ordinary life' (Ward, 1986).

Special projects

KT's Café is a café and gallery situated in a busy urban high street. It is funded by social services, and staffed at any one time by three workers (from a total of six) and three adults with learning disabilities (from a total of seven). The café is open between 10 a.m. and 3 p.m. every weekday. KT's is the brainchild of a deputy social services manager who wanted to develop alternatives to the traditional model of day care described above (Williamson, 1991). This manager wanted to create a setting in which adults could gain work experience, and learn basic catering and retailing skills.

Clients who are interested in gaining work experience and who have expressed an interest in the café come for a 4-week period during which they discover whether or not they want to work in the café, and whether the staff and clients want to work with them. They are then offered a contract for 6 or 12 months. At the end of this period, a joint decision is made as to whether they continue at KT's, or move into some other work experience or paid employment. Several clients who have worked at KT's are now in paid employment, one in Marks and Spencer's catering department, another at MacDonald's Hamburger Bar.

At the start of their work at KT's, clients are given a job description, a contract and a breakdown of the tasks they will undertake. In addition, each client has specific learning objectives to meet during his time at the café.

Richard, 29, has been working at KT's part-time for 2 years. He attended a day centre full-time before coming to the cafe, where he was described by staff as 'shy and withdrawn, making few attempts to communicate'. Despite having 'quite good understanding' he had difficulty making himself understood and was very self-conscious. When Richard first started at KT's, he would not come out from behind the food counter, and would only approach a customer at a table when accompanied by a member of staff. Three months later, he undertook all serving activities without any difficulty. According to staff, he could operate the electronic till and needed minimal help in finding the correct change. Richard had received speech and language therapy intermittently throughout his life. After a few months at KT's, he actually requested speech and language therapy because he said he was aware that he could not always make himself understood. His keyworker suggested that the degree of self-confidence and sense of self-worth that he had developed since he started working in the café had probably led him to make this request.

Residential settings

The principle of ordinary housing provision is a part of the principle of normalisation. People with learning disabilities have a right to live in ordinary homes of their own, enjoying the same domestic and recreational facilities as other members of society (Kings Fund, 1980; Humphreys et al., 1984; Taylor and Taylor,1986; Ward, 1988).

Community residential settings for people with learning disabilities may be funded and managed by social services, health authorities, charitable trusts or private individuals. There are no common characteristics in terms of size, setting or content: residential accommodation can be found in any and every kind of ordinary housing. Some establishments are staffed 24 hours a day, others are staffed during the day only, others have a warden living nearby.

Residential settings that are run by charitable trusts or by private individuals must comply with certain statutory regulations in order to be allowed to function. They are monitored by social service inspectors to ensure that standards of good practice are adhered to. If the inspectors are not satisfied that an establishment is complying with regulations, it can be closed down almost immediately.

The Brackens

The Brackens is a privately run home for nine adults (all men) with learning disabilities. It has charitable trust status. The house is a large Georgian house situated on the edge of a small village and has 20 acres of land, half of which is under cultivation. Each member of the household has his own room, and there are five communal rooms plus kitchen, utility room, office, bathrooms and shower rooms. There are various outbuildings, including a garage and a henhouse.

None of the men who live in the house have families who live locally; some have lived here for 15 years or more. Most of them visit their families once a year for 2 weeks when the house closes in the summer. There are six staff who work at the house. Ed, who has overall responsibility for the home, lives in a separate flat attached to the main house, with his wife and son. He has lived here for nearly 20 years, taking over responsibility from his step-parents who founded the Trust in 1968.

The daily routine is structured around household and garden tasks. Each resident has a particular responsibility for certain tasks, such as helping with cleaning, cooking, gardening, or looking after the geese and hens. In addition, the men visit the local town for shopping or recreational activities, although this is not a daily occurrence. They have limited contact with other residents in the village, although there are a number of villagers who have formed a group called 'Friends of The Brackens'. This small group of local people visit the house regularly, and occasionally take some of the residents for day trips or visits to the local cinema. The Friends also help to organise fund-raising events, such as the annual summer fete in the grounds of The Brackens. More recently, some of the residents have been asked to help cut the grass in the local churchyard. They are paid an hourly rate for this. Other than this, none of the men undertake any paid work or training of any kind. They spend the majority of their time contributing to the upkeep of the house and grounds.

22 St George's Road

22 St George's Road is a modern, detached house in a residential area of a small town. It was purchased by the local social services department in 1988 as a home for people returning from hospital to community-based accommodation. St George's Road is joint funded by social services and the health authority.

The house has five bedrooms, kitchen, dining room, two bathrooms, a sitting room which doubles as a staff 'sleeping in' room and a small office. Five residents aged between 25 and 49 years live in the house, supported by seven full time equivalent staff who provide a 24-hour service. All the residents have come from long-term hospital care. Some have high dependency needs, and continue to have challenging behaviour. Contact with families varies: two of them continue to have no contact, and the other three are able to see their families on a regular basis now that they live in the same locality.

The residents all receive some form of day service from the Wye Centre. They each take part in individual programme plans (IPPS) which help to identify individual needs. Each person's daily routine varies according to his or her individual needs, but in general the mornings are spent at the centre (followed by lunch at St George's Road), and the afternoons taken up with more community-based activities. These might include swimming, walking, gardening and working at the smallholding. Centre-based activities would include sessions with the speech and language therapist, occupational therapist or physiotherapist, or individual work on developing self-help skills and use of the computer. In the evenings, visits to the pub are not uncommon. No two weeks are the same.

Support for the staff at St George's Road is provided by the local community team for people with disabilities. Regular input, advice and training are provided by the team members. There is also regular support from the local special resource worker, a member of the special resource service for people with learning disabilities and challenging behaviours. This service was set up to support people with challenging behaviour and their carers in their own communities through formal input – assessments, planned intervention and ongoing evaluation – hands-on support when required, and providing staff with appropriate training and advice.

The differences between these two residential homes are not necessarily a reflection of their status as private versus public service establishments. There are many privately run homes that are very similar to St George's Road in terms of their organisational structure and day to day activities. It is equally the case that social services homes may be similar in organisation and outlook to The Brackens. The differences are also not wholly attributable to the variations in level of ability among the residents. In these examples, the residents at St George's Road had higher dependency needs than the residents at The Brackens, and to some extent the support services to each reflected this. However, there are many privately run homes for people with higher dependency needs, just as there are social services-run homes for people with fewer needs. What these homes do reflect are the differences that exist in terms of philosophy. The management and staff at The Brackens had no awareness of 'ordinary life principles'. Although they provided a caring environment for their residents, they did little to develop community awareness or provide opportunities for residents to exercise community-based choices. The residents' lives were centred almost entirely around the upkeep of the house. In contrast, the management and staff at St George's Road were committed to making ordinary life principles a reality for the five residents they were working with. The fact that these residents had high dependency needs did not prevent them from experiencing a wide range of community-based activities, as well as receiving help in developing self-help skills and community awareness. As with day services, it is differences in philosophy that determine to a large extent how residential services are delivered.

Community teams for people with learning disabilities in the UK

In many districts in the UK, services to people with learning disabilities are provided by teams of health and social services professionals. As a minimum, they include a community nurse and a social worker. (DHSS, 1971, 1980, 1981; NDT, 1976, 1985; Sines, 1985) More commonly, they are made up of a variety of professionals including clinical psychologists, occupational therapists, physiotherapists, speech and language therapists and sometimes psychiatrists, as well as a community nurse and a social worker. Typically, they share an office base, meet regularly as a team, adopt a democratic approach to decision making, and are committed to sharing skills and expertise. Team members are involved in every aspect of services to people with learning disabilities: assessment and planning, monitoring and training, supporting and guiding. A summary of the role of the community team is as follows (Abel, 1988):

1. To identify those people who have a learning disability, to assess and keep a register of each persons' current and future needs.
2. To document the local provision in terms of family support and relief care; residential services; day care services; leisure activities; voluntary services; educational opportunities; employment opportunities.
3. To be available to individuals with learning disabilities, their families

and carers, and to other professionals for consultation.

4. To structure their internal organisation so as to be effective in advertising their service; receiving and processing referrals; assessing the individual's total needs; selecting the appropriate services for the individual, operating specialist intervention when required.

One of the major advantages of such an approach is that there is considerable cross-referral between team members, and information about clients and their circumstances is readily available. When the team works well, there is also considerable mutual support available among people who have the same concerns and are often working with the same clients. The disadvantages seem to arise only when team members do not support each other, and there are personality clashes and disputes about the organisation of the team. This can lead to poor coordination of the team's activities and dissatisfaction among the team members (Wilson, 1979).

Community teams were first established in the 1970s as part of the initiative on developing care in the community (DHSS, 1971) and as more and more people with learning disabilities were moving from long-stay hospitals into community settings. They were designed to provide a service to people within a certain geographical area. The team's responsibility was to provide people in the community with whatever support services they required. These services were supposed to be individually led, in that each client's needs were assessed by the team and the appropriate services provided. One of the ways this is currently achieved is through the use of individual programme plans (IPPs), a system first developed in the USA for examining an individual's strengths and needs in every area of life (Figure 6.1) (Houts and Scott, 1975; Dickens, 1983; Brechin and Swain, 1986; Hitchins and Spence, 1991). Increasingly, the clients play the central part in deciding what services they require, and how they want to develop their skills and spend their time. Members of the team are involved in making these a reality.

The future of such community teams is uncertain in the context of a mixed economy of health care (Griffiths, 1988; DOH, 1989). In some districts, teams are no longer viable as individual professions such as psychologists and speech and language therapists establish their own contracts with health authorities, trusts and fund-holding general practitioners. In other districts, however, teams are being maintained on the grounds that they provide the most efficient coordinated service to people with learning disabilities in the locality. It may be that once the Community Care Bill (1988) becomes law, there will be more support for community teams. For the moment, all that can be said is that successful community teams can provide an excellent forum for providing a coordinated service to people with learning disabilities (Wilson, 1979).

HOW TO DRAW UP AN INDIVIDUAL DAY SERVICE PROGRAMME

1. Collect information: assessments, IPP needs/actions outcomes from goal cards etc.

2. Discuss with client and other interested people the content of the IDSP

3. Fill out IDSP sheet to complete list of goals as necessary.

4. Record the aims of the programme which can be in broad terms such as, 'I want a job'. Give each a number so that they can be identified.

5. Aims will usually fall into one of three categories which are appropriate for day service intervention: going to work; personal independence; use of leisure time.

6. List the goals you expect to be achieved in the coming year.

7. Give each goal a number to relate it to an aim, eg. 1.1, 2.4, 3.2.

8. Write goal cards, noting who will carry out the action.

9. Rule up review sheet to record monthly reviews of IDSP.

10. Note revisions made. When the original becomes unrecognisable rewrite the IDSP.

Figure 6.1 An example of an individual programme plan

INDIVIDUAL DAY SERVICE PROGRAMME

Client:

Keyworker:

IPP date   Review date:

Aims:

Goals:

IDSP REVIEW SHEET

Goal No	Date reviewed	Comments eg goal card issued goal card rewritten } give goal card discontinued } reasons

Figure 6.1 *(contd)*

Chapter 7
Issues in Service Delivery: II

Using Time and Expertise Efficiently

Whether the speech and language therapist is a member of a community team or not, one of the difficulties which she or he often has is deciding where to direct his or her time and expertise. In any geographical district served by a speech and language therapist, there may be as many as five day centres and 15 residential settings, all of which will have some individuals with communication needs. How do speech and language therapists allocate their time? How do they prioritise? What criteria can they use? There is no one solution or one right approach; different solutions apply in different circumstances. Some general guidelines are outlined below.

Stages in the introduction of a speech and language therapy service

1. Identify overall need for the service.
2. State professional aims and objectives clearly.
3. Encourage individual referrals.
4. Begin joint assessment with carers.
5. Identify specific individual needs against criteria for entry.
6. Decide on staff training strategy.
7. Decide on individual/group intervention.
8. Establish contracts.

The first stage is to identify the overall need for speech and language therapy services in each locale. This can best be achieved by visiting each centre and residential setting and meeting the staff and clients on an informal basis. This will be time-consuming, but it will be the most accurate way of determining the range of activities and events available to clients and what kind of day to day communication environment exists; management and staff's attitudes to, and past experience of, speech and language therapy; individual clients' interest in speech and language therapy. In the context of such informal visits, the therapist can begin to communicate to management and staff exactly what a speech and language therapy service might offer. How the therapist chooses to work will depend to some extent at least upon his or her own expertise and personal preferences. In some instances, it may be appropriate to state these directly to the manager of the centre or home. For example, the therapist's priorities might be:

1. Intervention with people with communication difficulties and challenging behaviour.
2. Intervention with individuals who have some awareness of their communication difficulty, and who have expressed a desire for change (e.g. Richard in Chapter 6).

Much lower on the list of priorities might be people who can make themselves understood, but who have 'minor articulation problems'. This will come as a surprise to many staff and managers, as they perceive the therapist as a person concerned only with articulation difficulties (Chaplin and Turner, 1988). By stating preferences and priorities at the outset, the therapist can establish the 'ground rules' for his or her contribution to the centre/home, and begin to dispel some of the myths surrounding speech and language therapy. Another approach might be to discuss with the manager the various criteria for entry into therapy described below. It is important at this stage to be as clear as possible about what speech and language therapy has to offer, without presenting too rigid or dogmatic a viewpoint.

The next stage is to determine more specifically which clients require speech and language therapy services. This might initially involve asking staff to complete short questionnaires on clients whom they think might benefit from the service. This can be achieved using the PCP , INTECOM or CASP Part 1 formats. It will help to establish what staff perceptions are and which clients they perceive as having communication difficulties. The therapist can use this information as a basis for deciding which clients she or he should assess on an individual basis. Occasionally, clients will ask to see the speech and language therapist direct.

In centres and residential settings where staff have had little or no previous experience of speech and language therapy, there may well be inappropriate referrals from staff, or a failure to refer those clients with more severe communication difficulties: 'Well, there's no point in sending her for speech therapy – she can't speak at all'. In some instances, there may be a more general lack of confidence in speech and language therapy intervention: 'We had a speech therapist here 10 years ago – she didn't do much for anyone'.

Therapists will also need to decide where the staff seem motivated to collaborate with them. If none of the staff groups in the day or residential settings seem to be showing much interest or support for any kind of intervention, then it may well be more appropriate to focus on staff training (Jones et al., 1992). This strategy is discussed below. However, if there are indications that staff seem interested and motivated, then a contract with them should be initiated.

Establishing 'Contracts' with Carers and Managers

Establishing 'contracts' is one way of clarifying the overall aim of the speech and language therapy service, and of ensuring that those involved are aware of the implications of their involvement. This is not a new concept, although it has received more attention among health care professionals since the advent of the buyer – provider model of health care (Griffiths, 1988; DOH, 1989; Klein, 1991; Scott and Marinker, 1992). In the past, contracts may have been of a more implicit nature, often taking the form of a verbal agreement between the parties involved. Today, they are more often written statements which state service objectives clearly and succinctly (Egan, 1990). This is viewed by many as a positive development for the client, carer or manager in terms of empowerment. In the past, clients and other service users might not have received a statement of intent or direction, or indeed any information on the timescale of the intervention. Under the new system, service providers are encouraged to provide this information at the start of the intervention, so that all parties know exactly what is involved. Some have argued that this limits the flexibility of a particular intervention but, if properly conducted, it should not do so. A contract between a client and a therapist (or therapist and carer/manager) should include the following:

1. An overview of the speech and language therapy service, what it can offer, what it offers to the day centre, residential setting, locality.
2. A statement about the nature of the client–therapist relationship, what the therapist expects from the client or carer as part of the collaboration.
3. A statement about the responsibilities of the therapist, for example, being at a particular meeting, carrying out regular assessments, reviews, providing support for staff, regular therapy for individuals, setting up groups etc.
4. A statement about the responsibilities of the carer or client in the intervention process, for example, being at a particular meeting, agreeing to practise particular exercises, being at all the group meetings etc.

This sort of contract can have a standard format which can be adapted to suit individuals or groups of clients. To be effective as a standard-setting device, the conditions of the contract will need to be periodically reviewed in order to determine whether or not it has been adhered to (CSLT, 1990).

Criteria for Entry and Exit from Therapy

Caseload prioritisation essentially involves deciding which clients require speech and language therapy, and on what basis. The demand for speech and language therapy services for adults with learning disabilities far outstrips supply (Whelan and Speake, 1974; Parker and Liddle, 1987; Enderby and Davies,1989; Noble, 1990) Wherever a therapist works, whether in a hospital or community setting, there will always be individuals and groups asking for his or her expertise. These people may not always know what they are asking for, and their expectations may be entirely inappropriate, but nonetheless they will ask for the service to be provided. Some of the difficulties associated with this mismatch between what service users expect, and what speech and language therapists can provide, has been discussed in an earlier section. Our concern here is with identifying first, the criteria that speech and language therapists use to admit clients for therapy, and secondly, the criteria they adopt for discharging clients. We have called these 'entry' and 'exit' criteria. An examination of such criteria was undertaken by Davies and van der Gaag (1992a). A panel of speech and language therapy 'experts' working with people with learning disabilities, selected on the basis of their clinical and/or teaching experience, was brought together for a 1-day workshop. They were asked, among other things, to identify the criteria they would use to make decisions about clients' entry and exit from therapy. The outcome of these discussions is given below.

Entry into therapy (Figure 7.1)

The experts agreed that entry into speech and language therapy is usually by one of two routes: either a request for therapy is made by a day centre manager, day care officer, teacher, or another professional on behalf of the client, or the speech and language therapist identifies the client's communication problem herself through screening assessments. Many speech and language therapists who are providing a new service, or resuming a service to a centre, will carry out a screening programme in order to identify the needs of the population. Whatever route is taken, entry into therapy is indicated if:

1. An assessment has identified a communication problem which exists in addition to the client's learning disability, or is associated with it.

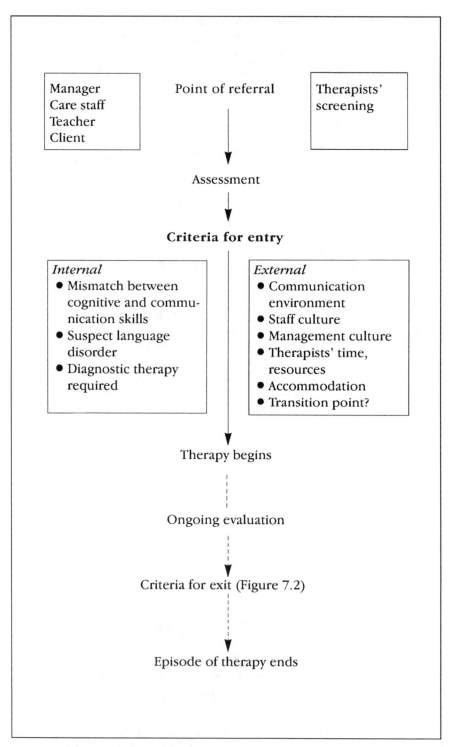

Figure 7.1   Summary of entry criteria

2. The assessment has established that the client is not making maximum use of his communication skills.
3. The assessment has established that the communication problem is rooted in 'environmental constraints'. These would include a communication environment which did not provide the client with sufficient opportunities to communicate (van der Gaag, 1989), or an environment where staff were not motivated to develop a client's skills, or work with the therapist.
4. The assessment has established that the client had some other specific communication difficulty, for example, non-fluency.
5. The assessment has established that a period of 'diagnostic' therapy is required. This usually means that a communication problem has been identified, but its precise nature and origins have not. Diagnostic therapy usually takes the form of an extended period of observation and assessment of the client in different settings.

In addition to these criteria, the experts agreed that entry into therapy would also be contingent upon:

1. A minimum level of support from the organisational structures and from the staff concerned.
2. Support from members of the community team, where appropriate. A therapist should not expect to work with a client without considering the client's communication needs in the context of his or her other needs, which may be being met by other members of the team.
3. The therapist must feel that she or he has something to offer the client, and has the time and resources to do so.

Finally, entry into therapy can occur at any 'transition point' in the client's life. Transition points can be negative or positive. An example of a positive transition point might be a move from hospital into a community residence. Another would be acquiring a new hearing aid, or new dentures. An example of a negative transition point might be the onset of poor health, either physical or mental, which would force a change in the pattern of intervention.

In the past, one of the areas often neglected by therapists in their initial approaches to working with adults with learning disabilities was developmental psychology as it related to adult development rather than development in childhood and adolescence. The literature on the psychology of 'being a adult' (Erickson, 1980; Egan, 1990) – of learning to adjust to the various stages or transition points of adulthood, of coping with new experiences such as birth, bereavement, loss, wealth and poverty, work and leisure, moving house, of learning more about sexuality, spirituality, social attitudes, stigma, expectations, health and illness – points out that these and many others are just as relevant to the lives of adults with disabilities as they are to the rest of the adult population. The tendency, however, was for the speech and language therapist to remain very much tied to the more familiar developmental concepts of childhood and adolescence, and not to focus upon these more relevant adult experiences when planning intervention. However, this pattern is changing, as therapists become more integrated into the organisational culture in which they work, and less dominated by the developmental approach on which they were nurtured as students. (For further discussion see Miller, 1990.)

There can be no doubt that the decision-making processes surrounding entry into therapy are very complex. This may be why so many therapists find it difficult to identify the criteria they use, and why they are somewhat reluctant to externalise the process to any great degree. However, the panel of experts was able to agree on the basic criteria which they felt to be appropriate to adults with learning difficulties. A number of points require expansion. First, we can conclude from the experts' observations that the organisational culture in which therapists find themselves will determine to a large extent who their clients are, how they plan their intervention, and when and on what basis they discharge them from therapy. This can mean the therapist may decide not to provide a service to a client with an identified communication problem if any of the following apply:

1. The management show no support for or interest in speech and language therapy services.
2. The day care officers/residential staff are not motivated to facilitate change in the client's communication.
3. The timetable does not allow for speech and language therapy intervention.

The danger in adopting these criteria is that no attempt is then made by the speech and language therapy service to alter attitudes and provide training for the management and staff. The importance of this type of input has been discussed above. Of course there are circumstances in which speech and language therapy services can provide a maximum amount of in-service training to very little effect, often because there is a poor management structure. This should not, however, deter therapists from ever providing this type of input at all.

Decision making is also contingent upon the individual characteristics and preferences of the client and therapist. The client's perception of his or her communication problem will be a major factor to consider. Therapists' interests should also be taken into the equation: they must feel that they have something to offer to the client (see Figure 7.1).

Exit from therapy (Figure 7.2)

The criteria for discharging clients from therapy may also, it seems, be determined by a combination of internal and external influences. Some clients are discharged relatively easily, according to one, or perhaps two, criteria. Others, because of the complex nature of their communication difficulties, may be discharged on several criteria. The experts provided the following list of criteria for exit from therapy.

A client may be discharged from therapy if:

1. The assessment indicates that therapy is not required. In most instances, the therapist will give advice to the referring agency, explaining why therapy is not indicated.
2. The objectives set at the beginning of therapy have been achieved, and so therapy is no longer required.
3. Appropriate support from the organisational structure is not made available, and so the original objectives cannot be met. This may mean a lack of necessary support from staff, management, family or friends. If this is so, the therapist may well need to redirect intervention into staff training.

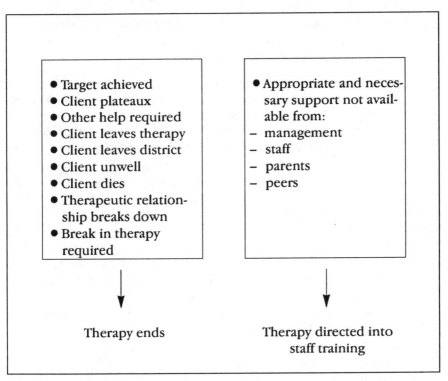

Figure 7.2   Summary of exit criteria

4. The client reaches a 'plateau' in therapy. This usually means that the client ceases to make any progress and requires a break from therapy. She or he may be reassessed at a later date, but is discharged from therapy on this basis.
5. The therapist requires a break from therapy. In some instances, the intensity of the therapeutic relationship and the nature of the client's communication difficulty may require the therapist to create some distance between him or herself and the client. Referral to another therapist may be indicated. For example, a client who has communication difficulties and challenging behaviours may require a period of speech and language therapy input followed by concentration on altering the circumstances within the environment that are precipitating or exacerbating the challenging behaviour, followed by a further period of speech and language therapy.
6. The client requires some other kind of professional help, for example psychiatric, psychological or medical, and is therefore transferred to another agency. This usually occurs when it becomes apparent that in order for speech and language therapy to be successful, some other kind of specialist help is necessary.
7. A personality clash between therapist and client occurs, making success in therapy unlikely.
8. The client chooses to discharge himself or herself from therapy.
9. Other circumstantial factors, such as when the client leaves the district, becomes ill or dies (see Figure 7.2).

The complexities of discharge criteria are compounded by the argument that people with learning disabilities are what some call 'developmentally disabled'. Their communication difficulties, along with their other difficulties, have been with them since birth, constantly changing, but ever present. They have not acquired them suddenly. They will, in one sense or another, always have learning disabilities, and will always have new targets to reach. They will therefore always require the kind of specialist help that speech and language therapists provide. Some therapists use this argument as a basis for continuing therapy over many years. They do not discharge clients, but instead place them on a review list for an indefinite period of time. A client may reach a target, and then be given a period to consolidate what she or he has learnt before continuing with a further period of therapy. During that period of consolidation, the client is put on review. This system is also favoured by many therapists because it does not involve any additional administration. No discharge forms need be completed and the client's name simply goes on to the review list.

The counter argument is, of course, that, however effective the therapist may be in using this approach, it constitutes an inefficient way of delivering a service. If therapists do not discharge clients when they reach the objectives outlined at the beginning of therapy, then there is no indication, beyond the therapist's own records, of the success of that period of therapy. There are counter arguments on a more philosophical level as well. An emphasis on the developmental aspects of learning disability is, to a certain extent at least, irrelevant to intervention with adults. The fact that people with learning disabilities have complex communication problems may have as much to do with the constraints on their communication environment as with any 'developmental' roots (Brenneis, 1982; Leudar and Fraser, 1985; Vogel, 1987; Sabsay and Platt, 1984; van der Gaag, 1989). Moreover, the emphasis on developmental aspects does not seem in line with the principle of allowing people with learning disabilities to lead 'culturally valued lives' (Wolfensberger, 1972, 1983), that is, to receive the services they require in order to meet their current communication needs. This emphasis on current needs fits more easily with an episodic model of speech and language therapy intervention, in which there is a definite beginning and end point, designed to address very specific objectives. When these objectives are met, the episode of therapy ends and the client is discharged. This is in line with the principles of goal planning (Houts and Scott, 1975), which have been in widespread use among the services to people with learning disabilities for some time.

Measuring Change

Having established guidelines for entry and exit from therapy, we now turn to the difficult issue of how to measure change and evaluate the success of intervention. It is now generally agreed that communication assessment must focus on three aspects: the clients' own communication skills, the carers' perceptions of the client, and the opportunities which the clients have to use their communication skills on a day to day basis. Whatever the client's abilities or circumstances, the speech and language therapist is interested in assessing all three aspects, and in setting specific objectives which will bring about positive changes for the client. There are various ways of achieving this. For example, Part 3 of the Communication Assessment Profile sets out guidelines for establishing priorities for change for each client (van der Gaag, 1988). ENABLE's Programme section has the same objective-setting principle (Hurst Brown and Keens, 1990) and the PCP 'shared action planning' provides another framework for this (Hitchins and Spence, 1991).

Measuring change involves setting specific objectives and then reviewing progress in those specific areas at a predetermined time. There must be a structure in order for change to be observed. Without structure, it becomes extremely difficult to evaluate progress in any recordable, definable, usable form. It is not enough to simply 'know' that someone is improving in some way: that knowledge has to be translated into a readable format.

In addition to identifying entry and exit criteria, Davies and van der Gaag invited the panel of speech and language therapy experts to discuss ways in which they would assess their clients' progress over time. The experts agreed on three general criteria:

1. There was a need to establish a baseline level of communicative functioning using a variety of subjective and objective assessment techniques.
2. There was a need to work with carers and other professionals on the development of the client's communication skills and on the communication environment.
3. In some situations it should be recognised that carers might be the primary 'client'. Therapists should expect to focus much of their expertise on work with the carer. They must therefore devise means of measuring change in this context as well.

Measuring change in the client's inherent communicative abilities is only one aspect of change: the influence of the environment and the carer must also be evaluated. What these criteria lead to is the principle that any measurement of change must be in terms of specific objectives set for a particular situation.

Measuring changes in the client

The panel of experts suggested a variety of ways in which to record progress in the clients' communicative abilities. A list of these approaches is given below. Assessments have been discussed in detail elsewhere in this book.

- Formal language and communication assessments
- Informal language and communication assessments
- Checklists of communication skills
- Video and audio tape analysis (pre- and post-intervention)
- Language sampling.

The experts agreed that, whatever assessment or combination of assessments is used, it must be applied at the beginning and end of the intervention if it is to be useful as an outcome measures.

Measuring changes in the environment

The panel of experts also recommended observing the client interacting with peers, carers and family where appropriate. Is there an optimal response by these individuals to the client? Is it appropriate communication? Is there a degree of choice within the client's day to day environment as to who he or she communicates with, and what about? What opportunities does the client have to communcate? Have they been targeted for change? Do they need to be?

Measuring the carers' attitudes and skills

Measuring the carers' attitudes and skills would also involve a variety of formal and informal measures. The experts recommended using pre- and post-training evaluation sheets such as those in the INTECOM package (Jones, 1990). They also suggested using informal observation of carers, and analysing video recordings of client–carer interactions. Calculator and Bedrosian's model for evaluating carer attitudes and skills was also recommended (Calculator and Bedrosian, 1988).

Agents of what change?

The measurement of change also depends upon how therapists perceive themselves. The argument for focusing on the extrinsic and intrinsic aspects outlined above is based on therapists viewing themselves as agents of change, not only in relation to clients' communication behaviour, but also in relation to clients' communication environment and their relationships (Mittler, 1984). If this is the model of intervention for therapists working with adults with learning disabilities, then it also directs the parameters of success of intervention. It is as legitimate to use a pre- and post-staff training questionnaire as a measure of change as it is to use a measure of linguistic ability. The challenge is to create such measures so that eventually they cover all aspects of speech and language therapy intervention.

In summary, the measurement of change can be achieved through the utilisation of simple recording methods. First it is essential to keep records at a macro level of the number of clients being seen, the amount of time spent with them, how many have achieved their goals and moved on, how many have not been seen etc. This provides therapists with month by month and year by year comparisons of the work that they are undertaking. Secondly, it is important to keep records at a micro level of individual clients' progress on specific goals, for example, checking how many clients have actually improved on measures of outcome, how many have stayed the same and how many have deteriorated over time. Finally, it is important to develop measures of carers' perceptions, which give an independent view of the clients' communication skills over time. These last two measures provide the therapist with a record of change in clients, carers and in the environment.

A Look at Staff Training

There is now a widespread realisation that the most important influences on the day to day lives of people with learning disabilities are those who spend most time with them, be they paid care staff, family or friends (Dalgliesh, 1983; Mittler, 1984; Anderson, 1987; Cullen, 1988).

The influence of the physical environment is, in most instances, secondary to the influence of the quality of the relationships that each person experiences (Landesman, Dwyer and Knowles, 1987). Cullen et al. (1984) found that people with learning disabilities living in a small hospital setting could expect to have a reaction from a member of staff to their behaviour on only 4% of occasions. Reactions from peers occurred on only 3% of occasions. In effect, this meant that for over 90% of the time the behaviour of these individuals would go completely unnoticed by those around them. Cullen points out that it is hardly surprising that such individuals develop unusual ways of behaving in order to attract attention. Although this type of evidence is not conclusive, it does support the view that, in order to change the behaviour of people with learning disabilities, one needs to change the behaviour of staff (Cullen,1988).

A parallel realisation among researchers and service providers is that the development of community-based services has meant an increase in the number and diversity of lay people who come into contact with people with learning disabilities. These may well be involved in making decisions about the lives of disabled people without having very much knowledge or understanding of their lives, much less any specific training. For example, they may make assumptions about people who do not communicate verbally, assuming that if they have no verbal communication skills, then they can have no understanding of verbal communication either.

This is not to say that the staff who 'looked after' people in institutions 10 or 20 years ago were any more informed, but there were probably fewer of them, and they almost certainly came from a less diverse and probably more medical tradition than many care staff working in community settings today. Community-based services in the 1990s are organised and delivered by managers from many different backgrounds, some with little or no hands-on experience of working in day or residential settings, and many with little or no training. According to a recent UK Social Services Inspectorate report (1989), only 13% of care staff surveyed had a qualification that related directly to their work with people with learning disabilities; 17% had trade qualifications (carpentry, metal work) and 18% had a teaching qualification. The report concluded that there was little evidence of any 'systematic staff training' in the community-based services surveyed. This survey did not include those community establishments which were run by health authorities.

The lack of any systematic training was identified by Mittler (1984) in his review of issues surrounding staff training in the learning disabilities field. He suggests that staff training must be the 'priority of priorities' in future planning, and makes a number of recommendations. First, staff training must be 'on the job' , it must be practical, and relate to the teaching of a whole range of personal and community living skills. Secondly, there needs to be a managerial commitment to staff training; staff need to have the support of their managers in order to be able to put their training into practice. Thirdly, there needs to be a greater commitment to record keeping which can actually chart a client's progress over time. This kind of record is an enormous encouragement to the care staff who are implementing a particular regime, because it actually demonstrates the success of what they are doing.

Mittler also suggests that there should be a strategic planning at the local and national level. He cites one training project in Manchester, UK (McBrien, 1981) as an example of the way in which staff training initiatives can be organised into a 'cascade' effect. Over 100 educational psychologists were trained in using behavioural teaching techniques on the condition that they set up similar courses in their own localities for teaching staff in schools. As a result, more than 1500 school staff were trained in the use of these techniques, and the materials have now been published as a self-teaching package. A similar 'cascade' approach has been used by Jones et al. (1992) in Somerset, UK (see below). For the majority of speech and language therapists working with adults with learning disabilities, the issues surrounding staff training are not so much whether to provide training, as how to provide training. In order to answer this, we need to look first at training effectiveness studies, which reveal something about which training techniques have been successful.

Cullen (1988), in his review of staff training, suggests that there was little evidence of the effectiveness of any of the traditional staff training techniques. In the short term, staff often say that they have benefited from in-service training courses, but in the long term there is little evidence that such training courses actually change the behaviour of staff towards clients. Ultimately, the effectiveness of training must be reflected in changes in the lives of clients, and not dependent upon staff perceptions of their knowledge base before and after training. The results to date are not encouraging.

Cullen goes on to observe that the majority of current training is geared towards one to one teaching techniques – hardly relevant to a staff group who spend so little time in one to one situations with their clients, largely because of the way the system is organised (Cullen, 1987). It is impossible to separate staff training from the organisational structures and management regimes which dictate to a large degree how people will spend their time.

A major review of staff training by Anderson (1987) in the USA is equally discouraging about the effectiveness of traditional techniques such as lectures and workshops. These methods are ineffective except in circumstances where they are supported by 'consequences for staff behaviour', such as giving staff more control over their own work timetables etc. These types of incentive are difficult to maintain over time, however. Anderson's review concludes that studies of modelling, role play and self-recording techniques are all inconclusive and do not provide enough evidence of their effectiveness. Others, such as the use of financial incentives, have proved successful in changing staff behaviour in the short term. The most successful training schedules, however, have included the use of feedback techniques, either videotapes or written or verbal feedback to staff.

Cullen's (1988) conclusion regarding staff training is that new methods must be devised and more empirical research must be undertaken to evaluate the effectiveness of different techniques. He suggests guidelines for staff training, which are based upon the characteristics of intermediate technology, a kind of practical, 'bottom up' approach, as opposed to a sophisticated, 'top down' approach. Training must be measurable in terms of its effectiveness, it should not be costly in terms of time and resources, it should be flexible, and it should be conducted on a small scale, preferably by local personnel. It should also be 'consistent with existing values and subcultures' (p.320).

One new system which may provide alternative ways of training care staff in the UK is distance learning, along the lines of the long-established Open University courses. It may be that qualification incentives, and individual learning techniques such as these, might suit carers who wish to develop their knowledge. The National Council for Vocational Qualifications (NCVQ) (1988) was established to develop such alternative routes to learning. It is likely that, in the near future, National Vocational Qualifications for care staff in day and residential settings will become available.

Before drawing some guidelines about staff training in relation to speech and language therapy, it is worth looking for a moment at carers' expectations of such therapy. A recent study of speech and language therapy services in six health districts in the UK (van der Gaag and Davies, 1992c) included a survey of 139 carers' expectations and opinions on speech and language therapy. This survey found that the majority of carers expected the service to provide them with ongoing support and training, as well as providing specialist input with particular clients. Of course, this does not clarify what kind of training was expected, but it did identify an expectation, which may not always have been prevalent among care staff. One might conclude that this sample of carers, at the very least, recognised their need for training. At best, they may have recognised the need for ongoing support from the speech and language therapist in order to be able to sustain the application of new knowledge and the exercise of new skills.

What, then, are the lessons to be learnt from the debate on staff training?

1. Training staff is important to, and necessary for, the success of any

intervention regime. It could be argued that training staff is no longer an optional component of the work of a speech and language therapist, but an essential, ongoing commitment. In order to develop the communication skills of the clients, it may be essential to first change the behaviour of the staff (Cullen, 1988).

2. The most effective teaching techniques are not the formal, 'one-off' lectures or workshops on 'communication'. They are the ongoing use of feedback techniques: the use of videotapes to look at client and staff interactions, the use of verbal feedback on staff use of particular therapeutic methods, the use of written feedback, keeping records of client's progress over time and discussing these with carers who have been involved in working towards particular goals with clients.

3. The success of any training initiative depends upon securing and maintaining the support of the management. As Hurst Brown and Keens (1990) point out, it is essential to establish this with the management prior to any training initiative. This might involve drawing up an agreement, both verbally and confirmed in writing before any training takes place.

4. The therapist should spend time identifying the job requirements of the staff, and design the training schedule around these. The tasks on which the carer spends most time should be identified. What does the job require? It is important that the training is moulded as closely as possible to the individual care staff, and the context or contexts in which they work. The therapist should be as specific as possible to the individuals involved, and draw on available materials and resources, but not rely solely on lectures and workshop settings.

5. The training should be as practical as possible, as relevant to the carer's everyday experience of the client's communication as possible, and as straightforward as possible.

Different Working Practices

There are as many ways of working as there are therapists. Below are examples which illustrate some of the different working practices that exist.

A model of good practice: staff training

The section above has provided some general guidelines on implementing staff training. For a further illustration on staff training methods, the reader is referred to the outline on the INTECOM training package (Jones, 1990) in Chapter 4. INTECOM provides a comprehensive guide to training staff in day and residential settings. The example below is a training schedule devised specifically for lay people involved in the lives of people with learning disabilities (Whitefoot and Tuck,1990; Errey, 1988).

Discovering communication

This training schedule was designed by Sue Whitefoot, a speech and language therapist, and Liz Tuck, a residential social worker with adults with learning disabilities. It was a course for 'friends, relatives or carers of someone with a learning disability', which was run initially over six 2-hour sessions spread over 7 weeks. Whitefoot and Tuck set up the training in response to requests from carers and friends of individuals with learning disabilities living in the locality. These carers felt they had little opportunity for learning about communication and how best to facilitate communication skills.

One of the strengths of Whitefoot and Tuck's approach was the way in which they made extensive use of feedback techniques such as video tapes, practical exercises including role play and brainstorming techniques, and practical assignments, such as profiling particular individuals. The format was not one-off 'lectures' (Figure 7.3) In addition, at the end of each session, the participants were asked to complete an evaluation sheet which gave them the opportunity to comment on the course content and presentation at each stage.

Whitefoot and Tuck also ensured that the course had the financial support of local agencies, which meant that participants did not have to pay for themselves. In the longer term , it may receive funding from health and social services and hopefully become incorporated into the National Vocational Qualifications system.

In their analysis of the participants' course evaluations, Whitefoot and Tuck concluded that the benefits of running a course for a mixed group of interested lay people were considerable. The participants learnt from each other's varied experience of living and working with people with learning disabilities. The course helped to demystify people's perceptions of professionals and professional jargon; it also helped to clarify practical aspects such as where local professionals could be contacted, and what jargon they might use. As a result of the techniques used, the course had a structure but was not formal, and allowed participants to get to know each other's views and to become involved in in-depth discussions. There were also advantages to having a course organised by a speech and language therapist and a social worker, who had different but complementary expertise to contribute. Finally, the participants themselves were very positive about the course structure and content, and were keen to attend the follow-up session.

One follow-up session was planned during the following months in

Week 1 *What is communication?*
Getting to know each other and the expectations of the
course

What is communication?
• active participation, brainstorming
• video and audio tapes to identify different aspects of communication

(Participants asked to write a profile of someone they know for
discussion in Session II)

Week 2 *Communication and the environment*
What is communication? – feedback on profiles

Trying to communicate in difficult circumstances, experiencing
'incomplete communication' – group participation – role play

Environmental influences on communication:
video and discussion

Week 3 *Communication continued*
Physical and social aspects (use of role play and discussion)

Choices/personal values: how do they influence communication?
Discussion

Week 4 *Breakdown of communication*
Personal values – feedback
Understanding 'understanding': difficulties
with understanding (use of videos)

Practical ways of checking understanding
What is pre-empting?

Week 5 *Changing relationships* – what improved communication
means to all concerned

General strategies to encourage expressive language

Communication aids – who for?
Augmentative forms of communication: growing up with sign/
symbol systems

Week 6 *Visiting experts*

Social worker for the deaf; the value of hearing aids (use of video
and discussion)

Specialist speech and language therapist: practical session on
communication aids

Final course evaluation

Figure 7.3   Discovering communication course outline (Whitefoot and Tuck,
1991)

order to allow more time to cover certain topics. These included more practical advice on hearing aids, more on how to encourage communication, how to use Makaton effectively, and how to work more closely together. All the topics were chosen on the basis of feedback from the course participants. The possibility of the group continuing to meet regularly as a support group was also discussed.

This type of course meets a particular need for individuals without formal training who wish to learn more about communication and learning disability. For many years it has been recognised that carers can be the most effective agents of change in the lives of the people they care for (Mittler, 1984). Courses like the one described above can give carers the knowledge and understanding – and the confidence – to become change agents in a way that no one-off lecture can ever do (Cullen, 1988).

Working with individuals

Karen

Karen is a 22-year-old woman who comes to the day centre every day. She has a severe hearing impairment as well as a severe learning disability. She had no intelligible speech, but communicated her needs through signs and pointing. She attended a residential school for the deaf before coming to the day centre, and it was there that she learned British Sign Language (BSL). Unfortunately, BSL is not used at the day centre, and her parents do not use BSL either. Karen was not well liked by some people in the centre because she was moody and prone to violent outbursts. Her keyworker referred her to the speech and language therapist, but when the therapist arrived to see her, Karen refused to cooperate. After some negotiation, Karen agreed to see the therapist if her keyworker was there as well. They decided together that they would work on Karen's ability to articulate the names of people familiar to her. The therapist and keyworker had used articulograms to give Karen visual cues for specific sounds, and rhythms (clapping etc.) to help with establishing correct syllable usage. Her keyworker made some miniature articulograms that Karen carried around in a credit card carrier to use as a visual cue when she needed one. In addition, the speech and language therapist and keyworker learned BSL. After 6 months of once-weekly therapy and daily practice with her keyworker, Karen was articulating the names of 20 different people, and using these spontaneously. As a result of this initiative, Karen also became more confident about using speech generally. She also became less inclined towards violent outbursts. The speech and language therapist said that Karen's success was due to her close relationship with her keyworker, and her keyworker's commitment to daily practice of her exercises.

Alan

Alan is a 27-year-old man who comes to the centre three times a week. He works in the local library once a week, cataloguing books and stacking shelves. He uses the local bus to get to work. He is currently attending a literacy course at the FE College, which he greatly enjoys. Alan lives with his mother, a widow. He visits the local pub regularly with friends, enjoys sport and being outdoors. His learning disability has been described as moderate.

At his last IPP, Alan asked for speech and language therapy. He said that he was having difficulty in making himself understood, and at times felt embarrassed by this. Where possible, he avoided conversations with people he did not know. A few months later, the speech and language therapist saw him. She found that he had particular difficulty with 's' clusters (words beginning with sl, sp, sw, sk etc.), and with 'ch' and 'j'. He frequently used glottal stops at the ends of words, which also made him difficult to understand at times.

Alan began having a weekly speech and language therapy session with the therapist. He learnt a new sound or sound combination every week for 23 weeks. At the end of this, Alan could produce all the 'ch', 'j', and 's' clusters in single word contexts, and had mastered most of them in sentences as well. All the people who came into contact with him commented on how much clearer his speech was. Alan's confidence in himself grew as a result, and he no longer avoided conversations with people he did not know.

The success of Alan's therapy had a great deal to do with his motivation to change. The therapist used standard listening and production techniques to develop his articulation skills, and placed great emphasis on the need for daily practice. She used diagrams to indicate correct tongue positions, which Alan found very helpful when thinking through how he would produce a sound. He always began learning a new sound by producing it in isolation, with vowel sounds, in single words and then in sentences. He had a book of exercises which allowed him to practise during the day and in the evenings. The therapist also used his literacy skills to give him a context in which to practise the newly acquired sounds.

What is interesting about these examples is that they illustrate that the once-weekly intervention model is not entirely without success (Jones, 1990).There are situations where this type of intervention can be appropriate. When an individual client is motivated to develop his or her communication skills, or when a carer is motivated to help a client to communicate more effectively, there can be change in well established acticulatory patterns.

Working with groups

A young people's group

This group was established by a speech and language therapist and carer in response to concerns about school leavers who were about to become users of adult day services. These concerns were shared by the local head teacher and day centre manager, both of whom had observed a few young people they knew becoming distressed and lonely during this period of their lives. The aims of the group were therefore to help ease the transition, to foster friendships, to develop new skills and to give young people the opportunity to learn about the choices available to them as adults.

The first stage of this initiative was to contact the parents of young people in the locality and ask them whether they would support such a group. There was unanimous support for the idea. The parents were given a short questionnaire asking them to comment on what they saw as the priorities for such a group. For example, they were asked whether they considered communication skills, assertiveness skills, social skills, information about work experience and further education important to their son or daughter. They were also asked what subjects their son or daughter was particularly interested in – fashion, food, music, sport etc. This questionnaire helped in planning the topics and activities of the group.

From this, a group of 10 young people aged between 17 and 22 years began meeting in the community centre for one morning a month. They took part in a wide variety of discussions and activities, including discussions with people who were already attending the day centre, and people on work experience and at FE college. The group went on visits together, and took part in a variety of role play and discussion sessions exploring different topics. Above all, they made relationships and friends, which many of them maintained after leaving the group. They had the opportunity to discuss particular worries or problems with the therapist or carer if they so wished.

A social skills group

Another example of group work with adults is provided by Cameron et al. (1988) They describe a group therapy initiative aimed at extending the clients' use of language and developing their interaction skills. They asked carers in the day centre to suggest individuals whom they felt might benefit from such a group. As a result, nine people met on a weekly basis one day a week for 8 weeks. The therapists were particularly concerned with developing 'initiation' skills, which were used in very limited ways by the group members. Consequently, opportunities to make choices and to communicate decisions to the rest of the group were given a focus in the group. Because the group met for a whole day, there were plenty of opportunities for this. The emphasis was on shifting the locus of decision making and control from the therapist and keyworker to the clients.

At the end of the 8 weeks, all the clients were judged by their keyworkers (subjective judgements by those who had not taken part in the group) to be initiating communication more often, asking questions and generally more confident about using their communication skills.

Developing this type of group activity is quite a common undertaking for the speech and language therapist. A group can provide a natural context for many communication experiences. It can also provide an ideal context for skills sharing. Specific techniques can be demonstrated to carers, who can then begin to use the same techniques in other situations. The therapists often finds themselves very involved in planning group activities, gradually working towards giving the carer more responsibility for running the group as it becomes established. Groups such as these are most successful if they are run over a predetermined time period.

Working with other therapists

The importance of the team approach in working with people with disabilities has been introduced earlier in the context of community teams. As a consequence of the growth of multidisciplinary team work in this area, therapists from all disciplines are working more closely than in the past, and are developing shared roles and perspectives (Bulpitt and Turner, 1988). One of the areas in which this development is very much in evidence is in collaborations with drama, movement, art and music therapists (Sherbourne, 1971; McIntyre, 1981; Kersner, 1987; Barnes, 1988; Shenton, 1990). With this increase in skill sharing, speech and language therapists are learning new techniques and approaches as well as contributing to the knowledge base of their drama, art and musical colleagues.

An example of such an initiative is reported by Kersner (1987), a speech and language therapist trained in the use of drama therapy. She set up a drama workshop for a group of adults in a day centre. The group staged one full-length play which was so successful that they went on to stage another. (Both plays were written by Kersner, and are now available from Alphabet books.) In her reflections on the success of the workshops, Kersner concludes that the most significant effect of such activities was in 'creating an experience which was shared by a community' (p.2). This had very positive implications in terms of opportunities for interaction and communication. Barnes (1988), another speech and language therapist who used drama in her work with young people with learning disabilities, expressed very similar views. She suggested that 'drama offers the therapist a stimulating and lively communicative medium through which to tap all aspects of non-verbal and verbal language' (p.2). McIntyre (1981) felt that drama's potential as a therapeutic medium was vast. It involves so many elements: movement, sensory awareness, mime, improvisation – all vehicles for self-expression and creativity. Perhaps over and above its therapeutic aspects, drama is also very good fun, very stimulating, and very different from routine, day to day life experiences. This is its major appeal to all of us, with or without disabilities. The growing number of productions by theatre companies run for and by people with disabilities provides a testament to this (Stange, 1980; Tomlinson, 1982; Freeman, 1988).

Collaborations with movement, art and music therapists are also becoming more commonplace in work with people with disabilities (Sherbourne, 1971; Levitt,1987; Shenton, 1990; Strong, 1991). Speech and language therapists are increasingly seeing these art forms as a medium for increasing skills such as sequencing, concentration and attention, as well as body awareness and spatial awareness. These therapies can contribute enormously to self-confidence and to establishing positive relationships, both of which are important to the development of communication skills (Laban, 1951; Sherbourne, 1971; North, 1972).

'Making communication a priority'

'Making communication a priority' was the title of an article which described an innovative approach to service delivery established by Jane Jones and her colleagues in the UK (Jones et al., 1992). This approach focuses on a 'total communication' strategy for adults with learning disabilities. Total communication essentially means devising an individually based strategy for 'the complementary use of signs, symbols and speech to enhance verbal comprehension, improve expressive ability and develop a form of literacy' (p.6). Jones et al. give an example of how such a strategy can be implemented by involving all the individuals who come into contact with the client on a day to day basis. By working together, therapist, client and staff devised a relevant vocabulary for the client, and then a symbol and a sign to match each vocabulary item. Rebus and BSL symbols were used wherever possible. Signs and symbols were taught using lotto games made up of a series of photographs. Signs and symbols were gradually devised for all the environments, people and activities that were part of the client's life.

In order for total communication to work, Jones and her colleagues devised an imaginative staff training project which was eventually implemented on a county-wide basis. They began by convincing health and social services management to commit resources to the development of the total communication approach for all staff. They developed a three-tiered staff training scheme, each with syllabus and certificate. The first comprised a 7-hour induction training package, which all staff in the area were required to attend. The second was a 3-day advanced course for staff wanting to learn how to develop their own symbols with their clients. Staff who attended these advanced courses could then attend a week-long course to further develop their skills. Having completed all three stages, staff would then become 'coordinators'. Under the local county council's policy, each establishment serving adults with learning disabilities is now expected to have at least one coordinator, who is responsible for the induction training for new staff members. There are currently 150 coordinators in the county. An extensive library of signs and symbols has been built up over the years and is available for general use.

There are three aspects of this approach that are important. The first is that it is driven by the individual's communication needs. The second is that its success depends upon the wholehearted involvement of the staff and peer group. Everyone (who is able) in the clients' environment is asked to learn the signs and symbols, and to make use of them in everyday communication. Every member of staff is encouraged to develop his or her skills and understanding of communication. Speech and language therapy resources are concentrated on developing the skills of carers. The speech and language therapists have adopted a consultant's role, a training role, and are engaged in very little one to one therapy with individual clients. Their skills are focused on detailed assessment and planning, and on empowering others by giving them knowledge and skills directly relevant to their work with clients.

The third aspect of this approach that provides important guidance is the way in which senior managers were asked to take seriously the contribution of the speech and language therapy services to the training of all staff. This assertive and confident attitude, in which the speech and language therapists impressed upon managers the importance of their role as trainers, was vital to the success of total communication.

Meeting local needs: hearing assessments

One final example which provides an illustration of successful intervention comes from therapists' work in delivering a hearing assessment service to adults with learning disabilities (Pinney and Ferris Taylor, 1989; Harrell, 1990; Terrell, 1991). At times it may be appropriate to focus on a particular area of need, such as hearing, which is often neglected in spite of its vital contribution to effective communication. Other specialists have drawn attention to this issue in the past (Nolan et al., 1980; Yeates, 1980; Miles, 1984). The example below gives a snapshot view of this kind of approach.

Pinney and Ferris Taylor (1989), speech and language therapists who were members of a community team, decided to concentrate their resources on screening the hearing abilities of all adults with learning disabilities living in their district. They suggested that hearing assessment for this client group warranted investigation for a number of reasons; first, that there is a higher incidence of hearing loss among people with learning disabilities than in the overall population (Nolan et al., 1980; Kropka and Williams, 1986; Yeates, 1989). Secondly, that the effects of hearing loss are frequently attributed to other factors, such as communication difficulty, an unwillingness to cooperate, or just the fact that the individual has a learning disability. Carers will often be unaware that the presence of a hearing loss can exacerbate any and all of these factors in very significant ways (Denmark, 1978). A carer who complains that a client is uncooperative because 'he just doesn't bother to listen' may not have considered that the client cannot hear what is being said.

In the light of these concerns, Pinney and Ferris Taylor established a screening programme for adults within the district. They used a number of methods: free-field audiometry using a Peters A22 audiometer (or in some cases a paediatric warble tone audiometer), the Kendal Test modified for use with adults, and a visual examination of the external and middle ear using an auroscope. They found that the majority of clients were able to cooperate fully on either the pure tone or speech audiometric assessment: only three out of 140 clients assessed were unable to do so.

The screening initiative confirmed earlier reports that there is a higher incidence of hearing impairment among people with learning disabilities than the population as a whole (see also Yeates, 1980; Brister, 1986).

Moreover, Pinney and Ferris Taylor found that a large number of the individuals who used hearing aids also had some form of external auditory meatus problem such as impacted wax or chronic otitis media. This has been reported by other specialists, notably Miles (1984) and Yeates (1980). An even more striking finding was that 36% of those assessed had no other form of hearing impairment besides external auditory meatus problems.These problems are in general not only curable but can also be prevented through appropriate aural hygiene.

The follow up to Pinney and Ferris Taylor's screening initiative was to ensure that the clients with hearing problems received appropriate help. Public relations and educational strategies were used in addition to following up individual treatments. For example, Pinney and Ferris Taylor spent time liaising with ENT staff, audiometricians and GPs, raising the profile of their clients and drawing attention to the need for regular hearing assessment and appropriate treatment. They also spent time working with carers, explaining the more practical aspects of hearing loss. For example, they provided clients and carers with help and advice on the use and maintenance of hearing aids, and the importance of monitoring aural health and hygiene regularly. They liaised with the hearing therapist and the social worker for the deaf on behalf of individual clients about the use of environmental aids, such as TV listening aids and vibrating alarm clocks.

Terrell (1991) describes a very similar approach developed under the direction of the audiology services. Her concern was also with providing appropriate assessment and follow-up services for people with hearing impairments. She gives some useful examples of individuals who used the service in her district. Two of these are described below.

Paul

Paul is a 27-year-old man who has lived in institutions for most of his life. He was known to have had a severe hearing loss from a young age and had been provided with powerful BW81 hearing aids. However, these were abandoned because he could not be encouraged to wear them. He has little understanding or use of verbal communication but understands basic Makaton signs. He has a history of challenging behaviour.

When Paul first came to attention, his hearing aids were tried and it was found that he reacted to music. Two new postaural BE52 hearing aids were introduced after a postaural myogenic test was administered and showed a 80–90 dB hearing loss. Paul was encouraged to wear the aids but with little success; he rejected them as he had in the past. His speech and language therapist then decided that a different approach was needed. She devised a careful programme of introduction to the aids, designed to desensitize him to wearing the aid through the following steps:

1. Cotton wool in one ear.
2. Ear mould only, without aid attached.
3. Ear mould with aid attached but switched off.
4. Hearing aid switched on at a low volume.
5. Hearing aid switched on at appropriate volume.

Each step was broken down further into short time periods which were increased in frequency and duration. Success was taken as achieved when Paul wore the aid at each trial without touching it. If he did touch it, it was removed until the next trial period. When the time periods were felt to be of adequate frequency and length at each step, Paul moved on to the next step.

After 6 months, Paul was successful in learning to use the aid. Each step took several weeks to achieve. Use of the hearing aid has had a positive effect. Staff have noticed a marked change in his behaviour: he is less frustrated, the number of challenging behaviours has decreased, he responds more to people and has begun to vocalise. One of Paul's aids has been changed to a more refined commercial aid, a Phonak PP-C-L, which will hopefully be of even more benefit to him.

Unfortunately, this positive change in Paul's behaviour was reversed recently when he developed an ear infection and could not wear his aids. His frustration and outbursts increased. However, once the aids were reintroduced, this situation reverted again.

Bill

Bill is 67 years old and has a severe hearing loss. He lives in supported housing, has a part-time job and is independent in most living skills. He understands most successfully through reading and uses speech to communicate.

Staff have worked hard at encouraging Bill to wear his BE52 aid, as he has great difficulty hearing speech without it. He has been very reluctant to wear the aid, but has been encouraged to do so for specific conversations such as planning holidays. Bill has also acquired a TV listening device, a flashing smoke detector and doorbell. The doorbell has allowed him more privacy, as he can now answer the door and staff no longer need to use keys to get into his home.

Pinney and Ferris Taylor (1989) drew attention to the variation in standards of training in audiological assessment and management in speech and language therapy training establishments in the UK. In general terms, they considered that speech and language therapists were well trained in the theoretical aspects of hearing, but had more variable expertise in the practical aspects. Speech and language therapists are therefore in a good position to build upon their understanding and develop their skills in this area.

There is certainly some question as to whether Pinney and Ferris Taylor and Terrell were adopting a role more appropriate to an audiometrician or a hearing therapist when they undertook these hearing assessments. Pinney and Ferris Taylor discuss this in their report. They point out that there is undoubtedly a need for screening procedures for adults, and in some instances the speech and language therapist may be the only professional who can coordinate such an initiative. Hearing therapists and audiometricians are in short supply, and sometimes may be reluctant to take on the responsibility for a screening initiative involving so many clients. This is also an area where the barriers to introducing the priniciple of normalisation can be most apparent. People with disabilities do not always have the same access to health care services as other members of society (Evans et al., 1987). Ordinary community services, such as the services of an audiometrician, may not be available to them in the same way (Flynn, 1989).

There is never any suggestion by either Pinney and Ferris Taylor or Terrell that speech and language therapists should be taking over the role of the hearing therapist or the audiometrician. Rather, the team should work together to provide the most accessible service for clients. Hearing assessments should not be an issue about professional boundaries but about meeting the needs of the local population in the most efficient and flexible way possible. As these studies have shown, the speech and language therapist can make an important contribution to this process, at least until the time when comprehensive community-based audiology services are established in every district (RNID, 1990). Once an initial screening exercise of this nature has been undertaken, then follow-up by community services is much easier and monitoring can become more efficient.

Working with Speech and Language Therapy Assistants

Evidence of the value of speech and language therapy assistants working in the UK comes from the work of Davies and van der Gaag (1992c, d,e) and van der Gaag and Davies (1992c,d,e). This research made use of observation and interview techniques, analysis of throughput data and pre- and post-intervention measures to evaluate the role of assistants working with three client groups: children, the elderly and people with learning disabilities. The results relevant to working with people with learning disabilities are reported below.

What do speech and language therapy assistants do?

The work of an assistant falls into three main categories: administration and preparation work, individual and group work with clients, and work with carers.

Administration and preparation

Speech and language therapy assistants can contribute to general administrative duties, such as photocopying, making phone calls, general filing. They also contribute to the preparation of therapy materials. One assistant who had considerable talent as an artist was able to supply the speech and language therapy department with a whole range of more appropriate pictures for use with individuals and with groups.

Individual and group work

The main use of speech and language therapy assistants in this area centres around giving clients one or more additional sessions of speech and language therapy during the week, so that more practice of specific targeted communication behaviours can be provided. Examples include signing and reading practice, listening work and dyspraxia exercises. The usual practice was for the therapist to see the client early in the week, and for the assistant to repeat the excerises later on in the week. Some of the assistants took the client out on 'community experience'. This involved visits to shops, museums, exhibitions, during which the assistant would concentrate on teaching a specific skill or skills in a real-life situation. This would reinforce the work being carried out in the day centre context.

Groupwork with the therapist and carer included signing groups and conversation groups, which focused on specific topics like shopping, foods, sports, music, clothes etc. Often the assistant and the carer would run these groups together without the therapist being present.

Working alongside carers

Speech and language therapy assistants also had a role in developing better working relationships with staff in day and residential settings. The very fact that they are not professionally trained means that they can help to break down barriers between the visiting speech and language therapist, perceived as an 'expert', and the carers, who often feel that they are in some sense less important, or have less status than the professionals. This divide is being broken down all the time, through in-service training initiatives, new joint ways of working, and better dialogue between therapists and carers. However, observations of assistants and reports by the carers themselves, suggest that assistants can become key people in the development of closer working relationships.

Key factors

The successes and failures of working with assistants appear to depend upon a number of key factors relating to recruitment, training and supervisory structures.

Recruitment

Choosing the right person for the job of an assistant is very similar to any recruitment procedure. Davies and van der Gaag found that the majority of people who are appointed as assistants were women aged between 35 and 55, who had worked in some kind of 'caring' capacity before, and who said at interview that they would like to work with people with learning disabilities. Previous experience of this work did not seem to be essential. The qualities which were considered essential were a high level of interpersonal skill, a positive and caring attitude and a recognisable degree of self-confidence.

Training

There seem to be a variety of different approaches to the training of assistants. They range from a 2-day induction course plus ad hoc training on the job, to a 4-week induction course, with structured observation periods, developing into an ongoing weekly training session lasting an hour.

The quality of an assistant's work would appear to depend not only on the suitability of the person for the job, but also on the training input. The speech and language therapy assistants who were not happy in their work were the ones who received minimal training and supervision from their therapists.

Induction courses

The exact length of the induction course will depend upon whether the assistant is employed on a full-time or a part-time basis. The recommended structure is a 4-week induction period, plus ongoing once-weekly training sessions (1 hour a week), and regular (3-monthly) day-long, or half-day 'refresher' courses on specific subjects as necessary. Ideally, the induction course should be run on a daily basis, with workshops, video presentations and lectures in the mornings, and observation sessions in the afternoons. This part of the training programme would be provided by the therapist in charge of the assistant, or in collaboration with a therapist designated as the Assistant Trainer for the district.

The content of the course should include:

1. *A general introduction to communication*: its component parts, its development and how it can break down; and also, principles of cognitive development, physical development, psychological development, and basic anatomy of the articulators.
2. *General introduction to speech and language therapy:* What is speech and language therapy? What do speech and language therapists do? Who do they work with? This should cover principles of assessment, diagnosis, goal planning and teaching techniques, specific communication and feeding programmes and how they work, audiological testing, augmentative and alternative systems, working with carers.
3. *Organisation of services*: How is the speech and language therapy department run? Who is the service for? etc.; organisational and administrative aspects; using the photocopier, filing and data collection systems; how the speech and language therapy service fits into

social, health and education services; health and safety at work.
4. *Learning disabilities*: how they arise – general introduction to the possible causes of disability; characteristics of learning disabilities – the relationship between communication development and cognitive development, related disabilities, the psychological effect of disability on families; principles of normalisation, the importance of attitudes, the influence of the environment; introduction to 'challenging behaviour' and why it occurs.
5. *Observation sessions:* these should include periods of:
   • General observation of the clients and therapist at work as well as in less formal settings.
   • General observation of other therapists working in other settings and with other client groups, e.g. community clinics, special schools, hospital settings.
   • Use of structured observation techniques: asking the assistant to look for specific behaviours, and record their occurrence within a particular time period, observing either real-life situations or video tapes.
   • Demonstration of specific teaching techniques, using real-life situations and video tapes, discussing examples of good and bad practice, rationale for using a particular technique etc.

At the end of the 4-week induction, the assistant should begin working alongside the therapist, continuing to use the observation techniques which she or he began learning during training. Gradually, the therapist should allow the assistant to work with clients, at first in a group setting, with the assistant giving help to one of the group members, and then one to one with the therapist observing. All such sessions should be concluded with a 'debriefing' session, during which the assistant is encouraged to analyse his or her own behaviour as well as the client's. Questions that are useful in this context include: What did I find most difficult about the session? What came easily? How well did the client do on this task? How well did she or he do compared with last time? This debriefing session will form the basis for the ongoing supervisory structure.

The most successful collaborations between therapists and their assistants included a weekly hour-long training session, which continued on a regular basis. The therapists and assistants would decide together what topics needed to be covered: sometimes this would be a teaching session on, for example, the use of signs or symbols, or the causes and characteristics of a particular syndrome. At other times, it would focus on a particular client, or on a particular problem that the assistant had come up against earlier in the week. In most instances, these weekly sessions were organised by two therapists and their assistants. A joint session was often more creative and less intense than a one to one session.

Supervision

Perhaps the least obvious and the most important element of supervision is that it is provided on a regular basis. Weekly training sessions, plus regular debriefing, allow the assistant and the therapist to maintain a clear idea of what the other is doing. Regular, ongoing supervision may not appear necessary once the assistant has become familiar with the routine, and is confident in what he or she is doing. However, the danger in not having a time in which the therapist and the assistant can discuss their work is that making time becomes more difficult for both parties, and it takes a crisis of some sort to bring the therapist and the assistant togther. Regular dialogue is a way of avoiding this.

Difficulties in working with assistants

1. Lack of accommodation. This appeared to be the major difficulty reported by therapists and assistants who took part in the study. Having another team member to accommodate in an already limited space was a source of frustration for many therapists.
2. Jargon. A few speech and language therapy assistants felt that they were 'left out' of staff meetings and special interest group meetings because they were not familiar with the professional jargon used by the speech and language therapists. This difficulty lessened the longer the assistants were in post, presumably because they became more familiar with the terms being used.
3. Uncertainties about the role of assistants. This occurred where speech and language therapists were relatively new to working with adults with learning disabilities, and themselves felt uncertain about their role. The responsibility for organising the assistant's work schedule as well as their own was a burden some of them would have preferred not to carry. In one instance, the therapist felt that she was having to look for extraneous activities which she thought the assistant could cope with, rather than working through her caseload priorities and allocating work to her assistant accordingly. This was clearly not a satisfactory arrangement for either the therapist or her assistant.
4. Finally, there was little evidence from the study to suggest that assistants will increase the throughput of clients during their first 12 months of working. Davies and van der Gaag (1992e) suggest that this may be due to the extra time which therapists need to take to train and supervise their assistants. This has important cost and effectiveness implications for the introduction of assistants. However, the possibilities for skills mix within the speech and language therapy profession in the UK are just beginning to become formalised and structured according to recognised standards (CSLT,

1991). In the USA and Canada, where support personnel have been used for some time, guidelines are already well established (ASHA 1980; CASLPA, 1989).

Part III
Future Directions

Chapter 8
An Integrated Model of Communication Assessment

Pragmatics and Linguistics: Is There a Dichotomy?

Having discussed existing assessment procedures and service delivery issues, we now turn to a model which is designed to complement current approaches to assessment and attempts to redress existing imbalances. One of the issues which needs to be addressed in this context is the perceived dichotomy between pragmatics and linguistics alluded to in Chapter 1.

Example 1

Situation: long distance flight London–Singapore. Lights go out and film begins to show.
A is sitting in aisle seat, Row 55, watching film.
B is walking down aisle, recognises friend in row 50, stops for a chat, blocking A's view.
A says: 'I am trying to watch the film. You are in my way and I can't see the screen. Please get out of my way!'
B gets down on his haunches.
Communication is successful: A's utterance means his intended message.

Example 2

Situation : as above *but*
A goes up to B and says: 'You are not made of glass, you know!'
B gets down on his haunches.
Communication is successful; it is achieved through the medium of language, but notice the discrepancy between the meaning of A's utterance and the message conveyed.

163

Example 3

Situation: as above BUT
A shifts in his seat, raises the back of his seat, cranes his neck, coughs, leans out.
B notices A's acrobatic exercises and gets down on his haunches.
Communication is successful in the complete absence of language.

Example 4

A: 'Did your treatment for stammering work?'
B: 'Peter Piper picked a peck of pickled pepper.'
A: 'How amazing!'
B: 'Yes, b-b-but th-th-that's not s-s-something I v-v-very often w-w-want to s-s-say.'
(From Sperber and Wilson, 1986, p.178.)
Communication is, again, successful; it is again achieved by the use of language, but can B's first reply be considered to be a case of verbal communication in the same way as in Example 2?

Example 5

Situation: A has been evicted from his apartment and is asked for the reason for the eviction, to which he replies:
'Well, a couple of reasons. They didn't – number one, they didn't fumigate or anything the building. They go, 'that's a brand new door there'. And they say – the guy in one-oh-two smashed the other door.'
(From Kernan and Sabsay, 1989, p.232.)
Communication is unsuccessful, because the grounds for the eviction are not explained, though, apart from the odd false start and hesitation, perfectly acceptable language is used.

All these examples show that 'meaning does not exist ready-made in the linguistic code, but is rather a function of the relationships between language forms, functions, and context, including the intentions of the speaker and the expectations of the hearer' (Wesche, 1983, p.42).

Everyone who has a fascination for language and communication is apt to ask, as the philosopher Searle did: 'How is it possible that when a speaker stands before a hearer and emits an acoustic blast such remarkable things occur as: the speaker means something; the sounds he emits mean something; the hearer understands what is meant...?' (Searle, 1969, p.3). Janet Daley referred to the same phenomenon in *The Independent*: 'As a novelist, I am constantly thankful for the fact that every English conversation has three levels of meaning: what you think, what you say and what you wish to be understood as saying.'

The history of linguistics is littered with different approaches that have attempted to explain this phenomenon. As we discussed in Chapter 1, various paradigm shifts have taken place depending on where theorists and practioners felt the focus of enquiry should be. This has often led to fiercely competing theories as to where the primary locus of the power of language lies. However, 'in the heat of controversy, it is sometimes tempting to overstate a position in order to press the opposition (real or imagined) into a frame of mind where the claims of a given theoretical stance will have to be taken seriously – if only to be summarily rejected' (Oller and Khan, 1981, p.3). This is what has been happening in the combat between the 'pure' and applied theories of language.

The starting pistol in the race between linguistics and pragmatics has been triggered by Chomsky's (1965) distinction between competence and performance. His stated claim that the proper subject of linguistics is the idealised native speaker's competence, irrespective of perfomance factors, has a very solid theoretical justification. But it set the world of linguistics ablaze. By invoking the notion of the idealised native speaker, Chomsky actually committed no greater crime than what every experimental psychologist does when controlling for confounding variables in order to study a particular behaviour. His biggest crime in the eyes of psycholinguists, sociolinguists and ethnographic linguists was that he had no intention of going further and studying how language interacts with various aspects of the communicative context. There is no reason, though, why that enterprise should not be undertaken by someone else. Opponents of Chomsky, in the heat of the argument, took a diametrically opposing stance and declared that language could not exist outside communicative contexts, and went as far as claiming that it is indeed the pragmatic aspects of language that constrain the structure of language (Bates, 1976; Gazdar, 1979).

Something very similar has happened in applying linguistics to the clinical context. After a period of experimenting with formal linguistic models and finding them disappointing, many speech and language therapists have turned to the so-called 'pragmatic' or 'functional' approach, to the exclusion of linguistics. There is, however, a great danger in seeing different focuses as being in competition with each other, namely, that in the race for primacy we may never get to the finishing line. It is perfectly legitimate for theoreticians to limit the focus of their attention to any one aspect of a multifaceted behaviour like communication. Indeed, it is sometimes necessary to treat the various components in isolation. At some point, however, it is essential to adopt a holistic approach and examine how the components come together to create an outcome. It is undoubtedly the case in language that the functional and formal aspects mutually influence each other, and neither of them can or should be ascribed the leading role.

So, a pragmatic approach should not be seen as replacing a formal linguistic approach, but rather the two must be regarded as complementing each other.

The Pragmatic Framework

Pragmatics has been defined in many different ways since the term was first used by the philosopher Charles Morris in 1938. He defined it as the study of 'the relation of signs to interpreters'. According to some views it is that part of the study of meaning for which formal syntactic and semantic theories have no explanation, and has thus earned the dubious nickname the 'dustbin' of linguistics. According to others it is the set of social conventions which dictate how, when, with whom to talk, and for what purpose. There are also more extreme views which regard pragmatics as communication 'minus' language. The one thing that all these perspectives agree on is that pragmatics has to do with communication, i.e. with conveying messages. We shall adopt a working definition, that is, define pragmatics as the study of how speakers and hearers interact in exchanging information in various communicative situations. Additionally, whereas we acknowledge the existence and value of non-verbal communication either as replacing or as accompanying verbal communication, we shall assume, in the spirit of Chapter 2, that in an ideal communicative situation the primary medium is language. Moreover, as a starting point, we should like to concentrate on oral language, though, of course, what we have to say applies largely to all the various signing systems which are based on language, too.

Communication as a multifaceted activity

When we are engaged in communication we are in fact engaged in a number of activities simultaneously. The four core participants in a communicative act are the speaker, the hearer, the intended message and the communicative situation. Let us assume, for the sake of illustration, that the communicative situation is given and more or less beyond the control of the speaker or the hearer. The curtain rises with the first activity, a cognitive activity, on the part of the speaker. Knowing the situation and the hearer, she or he formulates a message she or he itends to share with the hearer. The next activity is a bodily one, e.g. she or he physically turns to the hearer, fixes his or her eye gaze appropriately, may or may not gesticulate with hands, may or may not change facial expression. The third activity is encoding the intended meaning in the codes of the language. The choice of the form, whether to express the meaning as literally as possible or by some more indirect form, depends on what she or he knows about the hearer, on his or her own personality, on his or her perception of the situation and the purpose for wanting to share the intended meaning. She or he then engages in a further physical act, namely making the utterance audible, i.e. producing the acoustic blast which Searle referred to. She or he controls the volume, the tone and various other physical aspects of the sound production. Presumably all along she or he is engaged in the cognitive activity of self-monitoring.

The following acts are performed by the hearer: she or he perceives the sound blast; as she or he does so she or he may or may not engage in some bodily movement, such as turning the head to the speaker, directing the eyes on the speaker etc. She or he then engages in the activity of decoding the literal meaning of the speaker's utterance. This is followed by the activity of making inferences on the basis of his or her knowledge of the speaker, of the situation and of the literal meaning of what she or he has just heard. Normally, the next activity is some tangible reaction from the hearer. Whether there is tangible reaction or not, it is more than likely that some form of further cognitive activity is evoked in the hearer. If it is tangible as well, it can be bodily movement with or without accompanying language. If language follows, of course the hearer becomes speaker and vice versa, and the whole cycle begins again. Alternatively, the original speaker may restart the cycle. It is important to stress that, although some sequencing of these activities is inevitable, some take place concurrently. Although, no doubt, we all know that this is precisely what happens when we communicate, it is worth detailing the particular moves. First, it is the totality of these that make up the study of pragmatics. Secondly, breakdown can occur at each and every move, with more or less catastrophic effects, and thirdly, these are the areas that various pragmatic profiles concentrate on.

In order to study communicative behaviours systematically, it is possible to organise these various moves into a number of main parameters, to provide a pragmatic framework. These are:

1. Context.
2. Type of message.
3. Organisation of exchange of information.
4. Non-linguistic communicative behaviour.
5. Presupposed knowledge.

We shall discuss these in some detail and make recommendations as to which components may need to be assessed. We do this, however, with the proviso that it is unlikely that all of our recommendations are appropriate or relevant for all clients and that clinicians therefore need to make the decision for each individual as to which particular parameter of the following pragmatic framework needs investigation.

Context

In Chapter 2 we characterised context as being made up of the communicative situation – i.e. the temporal, spatial and social setting – the medium of communication and the communication partners. More often than not, the social setting is given. This is likely to determine the place and time of the communicative event, the medium of communication and, to some extent, the relationship between the communication partners. However, nothing in a communicative event is ever immutable. A change in one component might well modify the others. The context is crucial in determining the type of message to be conveyed, the way in which the message is formulated and organised, the paralinguistic and non-linguistic behaviours and the knowledge that must be presupposed. It follows from this that communication can only be successful if both speaker and hearer perceive the nature of the context appropriately. Therefore we suggest that *the client's ability to judge the nature of context may need to be assessed.*

It also follows that different contexts have different implications for a client's communicative behaviour. Therefore we suggest that *assessments of communicative behaviour be undertaken in a number of different contexts,* namely the ones in which the client is most likely to participate.

Type of message

This refers to the speaker's communicative intentions. It includes the topics that communicative events are about and the purposes for which communication takes place. In Chapter 2 we provided some indication as to the nature and range of possible topics. We can only reiterate the fact that it is impossible to give a complete list of these, and that any classification is problematic. Everyone who undertakes the assessment of a client's communication is able to identify what the topic of a conversation is about. The assessor can also select a range of different topics that are relevant for the client. However, as different topics can have different implications for a client's communicative behaviour we suggest that *the range of topics a client is capable of communicating about both as speaker and as hearer may need to be assessed,* and that *in an assessment, the assessor should vary the topics of communication.*

There are several taxonomies that can classify the various purposes of communication. As in the case of topic classification, none of these attempts is entirely sucessful in that probably none of them is definitive or exhaustive. The boundaries between categories are often fuzzy. For example, when is a request an order? Classification and subclassification can probably be carried on ad infinitum until they become virtually useless. One commonly used, although not universally accepted, framework is based on Searle's speech act theory (Searle, 1969, 1976). He suggests that there are five kinds of basic communicative functions:

1. Representatives: these commit the speaker to the truth of the expressed proposition (e.g. asserting, concluding etc.)
2. Directives: these are attempts by the speaker to get the hearer to do something (e.g. requesting, questioning etc.)
3. Commissives: these commit the speaker to some future course of action (e.g. promising, threatening etc.)
4. Expressives: these express a psychological state (e.g. thanking, apologising, welcoming etc.)
5. Declarations: these effect immediate changes in the institutional state of affairs (e.g. declaring war, firing from employment etc.) (adapted from Levinson, 1983)

Needless to say, there is no need to insist on such classification. It is essential, however, that speakers and hearers should be capable of both expressing and recognising a wide range of functions, as well as adopting them appropriately to context and partners. Therefore we suggest that *the range of communicative functions a client expresses and is capable of recognising may need to be assessed,* and that *the appropriacy or otherwise of the client's use of these be evaluated.*

Organisation of exchange of information

This parameter refers to the linguistic organisation of some intended message on the one hand, and to the way the communicative interaction is structured, on the other.

First, we need to make a distinction between explicit and implied messages. We can go back to our examples at the beginning of this chapter. In Example 1, the linguistic meaning completely coincides with the intended meaning. This is a clear illustration of an explicit message: in Grice's term, an explicature (Grice, 1975). In Examples 2, 3 and 4 the relationship between what is expressed and the intended message is not so straightforward. The utterance 'You are not made of glass' means literally that the person addressed has not been manufactured out of glass – something he is probably well aware of. His reaction, however, shows that he was able to infer the implied message. The various bodily gestures in Example 3 are in themselves meaningless: there is a range of possible interpretations, but given the context, and given that B made the assumption that A is behaving in a strange manner for a particular purpose, again he was able to infer the implied message. In Example 4, the recital of a well-known tongue twister clearly did not mean to inform A about Peter Piper's action, but, served as an illustration of how the therapy was progressing. In the knowledge of the context, A was able to infer an implied message. According to Grice's definition, all information not explicitly derivable from the literal meaning of an utterance is an 'implicature'. Normal everyday conversation usually contains a plethora of implicatures. The English language is particularly rich in so-called 'idiomatic expressions' where the literal meaning of the expressions is divorced from the message they convey. For example the expression: 'Pull your socks up' is ambiguous between its literal meaning and its idiomatic meaning: 'Make an effort'. Only by appreciating the context is it possible to know which one was meant. In addition to idiomatic expressions, many words have both a literal and a metaphorical meaning. Also, speakers often opt for expressing their meanings in indirect forms to add humour, emphasis, or to give some emotional colouring to their message. In these cases hearers can normally make the right inferences by considering the context, knowing the speaker and relying on their knowledge of the world. An oblique statement can give rise to quite a number of implied messages. For example, in the following exchange:

A: 'Do you walk to work?'

B: 'Only animals walk, human beings have cars',

A, knowing that B is not an animal, can infer the implied message: 'no'. But B's choice of response gives rise to a number of further messages:

1. B does not like walking.
2. B probably has a car at his disposal.
3. B likes driving.
4. It's no use asking B on a hiking holiday.
5. If B's car breaks down, he probably stays at home.
6. B does not mind polluting the environment.
7. B is a selfish so and so.
8. B is flippant/likes to be entertaining etc., etc.

What is important to note is that there is a continuum of cases from those implicatures the speaker specifically wanted to convey, through those that were intentionally hinted at, to those the speaker never intended. The difference between explicatures and implicatures is that the latter are open to negotiation, whereas the former are guaranteed by the linguistic form. It is an essential component of speakers' communicative competence that they are able to produce as well as interpret implicatures. Therefore we suggest that *a client's ability to produce and to interpret indirect messages may need to be assessed.*

According to Grice, there are principles that guide the way in which we organise our messages. These he termed conversational maxims. These have to do with the amount, the quality, the style and the structuring of utterances. The four maxims are:

1. The maxim of quantity, i.e. say as much as is needed, neither more nor less;
2. The maxim of quality, i.e. say only things that you believe to be true;
3. The maxim of manner, i.e. be brief, orderly, avoid vagueness and ambiguity;
4. The maxim of relevance, i.e. say only things that are relevant.

These are supposed to specify what speakers need to do to make their conversations maximally effective. They can be flouted systematically for specific purposes, such as for humour, for misleading etc., and speakers and hearers base their inferences of implied messages on these maxims. Sperber and Wilson (1986) claim that their principle of relevance subsumes these maxims, and that there is neither need nor theoretical justification to give these principles a special status to the exclusion of a number of others which also play a part in our ability to comprehend intended messages. Briefly, the principle of relevance states that speakers always formulate their utterances in a way that it is most relevant to the hearer. This, of course, implies that relevance is measurable. Sperber and Wilson, do in fact, suggest a measure for it, which consists of two parts:

1. An utterance is as relevant as it is informative, where an utterance is informative to the extent that it enlarges the hearer's knowledge of the world.
2. An utterance is as relevant as is economical for the hearer to process it.

The two measures interact and in an ideal communicative act the two are finely balanced. Examples 1–4 above are all equally relevant by the first measure but differ in the degree of relevance depending on how easy B found it to process them, i.e. how easy it was for him 'to get the message' by the second measure above. The responses in Example 5 fail on both measures because they are not informative, and it is difficult to work out what message was being conveyed.

We can adopt this principle as a useful way of evaluating the effectiveness of a communicative act, and as Grice's maxims clearly form part of it we suggest that the *client's communicative abilities be assessed from the point of view of relevance, with particular reference to the Gricean maxims*.

Another aspect of the way in which we organise our communication has to do with the type of style or register we use. As native speakers we have available to us a number of different styles, from formal to informal, with subtle shades of difference encoded in the vocabulary, in the syntactic form and the phonology of utterances. Figure 8.1 illustrates this nicely.

The ability to choose the right style is as much part of communicative competence as the ability to choose what we say. Therefore, we

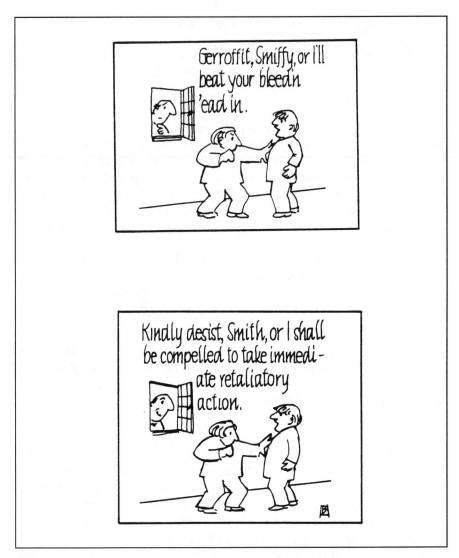

Figure 8.1

suggest that *a client's ability to modify his or her style according to context and participants may need to be assessed.*

Communicative events, of course, consist of a series of exchanges. Within any one exchange there may well be several utterances. In order to maintain the integrity and continuity of such exchanges, there are a number of linguistic and non-linguistic devices available to both speaker and hearer. The continuity can be 'explicit' or 'implicit'. If it is explicit it is assured by overt linguistic markers. These serve the double purpose of creating discourse cohesion and minimising processing effort. They comprise phonological, syntactic and lexical elements. For example, prosodic features such as volume, stress, intonation and duration are used for initiating a turn, introducing a new topic, signalling the intention that the speaker intends to 'carry on', or yielding a turn (Crystal, 1969). Contrastive stress can signal a difference between given and new information. The same distinction can be signalled by different syntactic structures. So, for example, if a speaker asked the question: 'How much rent do you pay for your room?' It would be as inappropriate to reply: 'I *pay* £40 per week' with contrastive stress on 'pay' as it would be to say: 'It is for my room that I pay £40'. The first is for phonological, the second for syntactic reasons, as both the exaggerated stress and the cleft construction, i.e. the use of the 'it is X that ...' formulation rather than the more neutral subject–predicate construction serve the purpose of introducing new ideas. Yet it is obvious from the question that it is precisely these two pieces of information that the original speaker had, or at least, assumed.

Another syntactic device is the so-called nominalisation to refer back to some event or state. For example, in the sentences: 'The horse jumped the highest fence. His jump delighted the audience', the first instance of the word 'jump' is a verb to express an action, whereas the second one is a noun to refer back to the same action. Halliday and Hazan (1976) describe a number of these lexical devices as cohesive ties, such as the use of conjunctions: 'and', 'but', 'so', 'therefore', 'however', 'also', or the use of anaphora to refer back to some entity, state or event. Anaphoric devices can be the use of co-reference, in other words referring to the same thing by another term, e.g. 'Mozart' – 'Viennese composer'; substitution by some pronominal form, e.g. 'Mozart' – 'he'; ellipsis, i.e. omitting to mention a term twice, e.g. 'Mozart was born in 1796 and was famous by the age of 5'; and lexical association, e.g. 'I like Mozart. Music is my favourite pastime' (Halliday and Hazan, 1976). There is no space here for giving a more detailed account of the precise nature and the full range of linguistic indicators of discourse cohesion. The reader is advised to turn to the works cited above for further details. However, since the absence of some of these devices can mean that conversations fall apart, we suggest that a *client's ability both to use these devices and to understand their import may need to be assessed.*

When it comes to implicit continuity there are no overt linguistic markers. Rather, the hearer must make inferences. We shall be dealing with inferences in more detail later in this chapter.

Structuring communicative interactions: conversation

Everything we have said about the linguistic organisation of communication applies to all types of discourse, be it a lecture or a conversation between two or more partners. In this book we are mainly concerned with conversation rather than any other form of communication. In addition to those features that ensure discourse cohesion and cohesiveness, there are a number of organisational characteristics that are peculiar to conversational exchanges. Some of these characteristics have to do with the so called 'local' management of the exchanges, whereas others relate to the overall, global organisation. Of the local ones we will deal with two which seem to be most relevant: turn taking and adjacency pairs.

Turn taking

What makes a conversation different from, say, a lecture is the expectation that two or more speakers 'take the floor' in turn. There are conventions which may differ in different cultures about how a speaker shows that he or she is yielding his or her turn and offers it to the conversational partner(s). This may be achieved by such overt linguistic markers as a question followed by some address term, e.g. 'And what do you think, John?' or a tag question with or without a following address term, e.g. 'He didn't look very anxious, did he (John)?' If an address term is used then the speaker has clearly selected who should take the next turn, and in this case there is an 'obligation' on the hearer to take over the turn. If no address term is used and there is more than one participant in the conversation, then one of these may self select after an appropriate silence. If no overt marker was used by the speaker at all, then after a short pause he or she may decide to resume the turn and carry on speaking. These conventions can be violated either inadvertently or on purpose to achieve some communicative effect. The violations can take the form of not waiting for the appropriate pause, leading to an overlap between two turns. If this was inadvertent, then one or the other of the turn initiators will normally yield his or her turn to the other. If it was done on purpose, then we talk of a deliberate interruption, which is often accompanied by slightly higher volume and slowed articulation. Another form of violation occurs when the selected speaker does not respond promptly and allows too much time to elapse, leading to gaps in the conversation. This can also be inadvertent or purposeful. If it is purposeful it is communicative, in that it yields possible messages, such as uncertainty, embarrassment, a wish to be impolite, expression of superiority etc.. The ability to signal the end of one's turn and the ability to respond to this signal are very basic components of communicative competence, and the lack of them can lead to serious problems in conversational communication. Therefore we recommend that *a client's turn taking strategies may need to be assessed.*

A more detailed account of the rules of turn taking can be found in Sacks et al. (1974) and a useful summary in Levinson (1983).

Adjacency pairs

If a conversation is to remain cohesive, then the contents of successive turns must clearly be related to each other in some way. Typically, the nature of a turn determines the nature of the response. It is in this sense that we are talking of adjacency pairs, which, like turns, are regarded as fundamental units of conversations. For two turns to be regarded as adjacency pairs a number of conditions need to be fulfilled. They must be adjacent; produced by different speakers; ordered as first part and second part; of a certain type, so that a particular first part requires a particular second, e.g. offers require acceptances or rejections, greetings require greetings, and so on (Levinson, 1983).

An example of a very simple, well ordered conversation fulfilling the above conditions would be in the context of a someone (A) knocking on someone's (B) door:

A: 'Hello'	(Greeting)
B: 'Hello'	(Greeting)
A: 'Would you like to make a contribution to the WWF?	(Request)
B: 'No, I have already done so.'	(Reject)

However, conversations are rarely quite so simple, and several further adjacency pairs may intervene between members of a pair; for example, in the context of a young man in a wine bar:

A: 'May I have a glass of white wine?'	(Question 1)
B: 'Are you over 18?'	(Question 2)
A: 'Yes.'	(Answer 2)
B: 'Do you want it chilled?'	(Question 3)
A: 'Yes, please.'	(Answer 3)
B: 'Here you are.'	(Answer 1)

In both of the above examples the various turns, whether strictly adjacent or containing nested pairs, are clearly contingent on one another. As in the case of turn taking, in adjacency pairs too speakers may violate the above conventions, either inadvertently or purposefully, with particular implied messages in mind. For example in the following exchange between a mother and child:

Child:	'Mummy can we go to the safari?'
Mother:	'Can we go to the moon?'

The type of response provided by the mother is not the most prototypical one, in that she responded to a question, with another question; moreover, the content of her response is not immediately related to the content of the question. But there is a strong implication that the answer is 'no' and the message will be conveyed successfully if the child is able to make the necessary inferential steps, first that it is impossible for them to go to the moon; and secondly that mother's only reason for talking about the moon is because it is somehow related to the child's question. The only relationship conceivable is the possibility or otherwise of going to either the safari or the moon, therefore, as the moon is impossible, so must be the safari!

It is much more difficult to find the same kind of contingency between the following two utterances:

A: 'Did you enjoy your dinner?'
B: 'My favourite programme is "Neighbours".'

Although it would be possible to find some communicative reason for B's reply in very special circumstances, (such as, he would rather change the subject because he did not enjoy dinner but does not want to say so explicitly) this kind of exchange is probably an example of inadvertent violation of conventions applying to adjacency pairs. It could be because B did not hear A's question; because he heard it but did not understand it; because he is not familiar with the conventions for well formed conversational exchanges, and so on. In other words, this could well be an example of a communicative disorder.

The exact mechanisms for maintaining smooth cohesiveness in conversational exchanges, beyond some of the tentative conventions we have mentioned, are still a matter of investigation, but here again Sperber and Wilson's (1986) relevance theory can be usefully applied. In other words, the baseline is that the speaker is trying to be maximally relevant. Therefore, any violation of the prototypical conventions indicates either additional implied messages, or a disorder. We suggest that *a client's ability to provide the right type of second member of an adjacency pair, as well as the degree of its relevance, may need to be assessed.*

There are a number of properties that characterise the overall organisation of a conversational exchange. These apply more to social discourse than to the relatively institutionalised short exchanges, such as requests for and supplying of information or services, or a simple offer and acceptance or refusal etc., although these can also contain some of the conventions. Typically, social discourse consists of quite a number of turns. Its structure can be seen as starting with an opening section, followed by various turns during which a topic is initiated, maintained, developed, changed and terminated. There can be a number of repairs in order to clear misunderstandings, clarify mis-hearings or non-hearings or to confirm correct understanding. After the last topic has been terminated there normally follows a closing-off section.

The opening section may start with an address term followed by some kind of introductory expression whose sole function is to signal the speaker's wish to start a conversation. For example:

A: ' Bobby, have you heard the latest?'
or
A: 'Maggie, I wonder if I could interrupt you'
or
A: 'Steve, do you want me to tell you what happened?'
etc.

The opening section is followed by a first topic which, by its very nature, is unconstrained by any previous turn. The following topics and turns are, by contrast, constrained in ways that we dealt with earlier under adjacency pairs.

The maintenance and development of the same topic are guaranteed by the various cohesive devices we have already spoken of. Changing and terminating a topic is often signalled by various linguistic markers. These can be quite overt, e.g. 'what you said reminds me of ...' or 'let me tell you about something else' or 'well, that was that' or 'what else can one say' etc. Even where new topics are introduced it is normal to maintain some kind of link with the previous ones, although topic jumps can also occur. The smooth running of the conversational exchange may be interrupted by so-called repairs when a speaker makes a mistake or hesitates. Repairs can be either self repairs or initiated by the partner(s). Self repairs are either repetitions or self corrections, often preceded by a short pause, with or without some noise such as 'ehm' etc. Partners may initiate repairs by direct questions, such as 'what', 'I beg your pardon' or by a puzzled look, or an over-lengthy pause as a response. The closing-off section can be quite elaborate in that the speaker initiates it by signalling that she or he wishes to terminate the exchange, which is responded to by the partner. It requires quite a delicate piece of social interaction and it is essential that both parties should wish to terminate the conversation. It can start with some kind of closing topic, such as arranging some future meeting, which is then followed by so-called 'passing terms', e.g. 'OK', 'so...' etc., finally concluded by terminal elements like 'bye-bye', 'see you' etc.

There are no hard and fast rules for the global organisation of conversations and individuals can adopt quite idiosyncratic devices to deal with the various stages of an exchange. Although some of them are of elementary importance to maintain polite social relationships, others are largely dependent on individual temperaments, which themselves are often dependent on the situation one finds oneself in, on self esteem, on emotional or physical state, not to mention general cognitive abilities. The ability or willingness to initiate, maintain, change or terminate topics may be useful to observe in a number of different settings with communication-disordered clients, if only to establish what kind of context encourages them to communicate and what hinders them, but we do not think that these need to be rigorously assessed. The more socially oriented conventions in maintaining the overall structure are perhaps of more significance. As Levinson (1983, p.321) puts it: 'Participants are constrained to utilize the expected procedures – not (or not only) because failure to do so would yield 'incoherent discourses' but because if they don't, they find themselves accountable for specific inferences that their behaviour will have generated.' For example, too slow or too fast termination of a conversational exchange may lead to unwelcome inferences regarding social relationships. Our suggestion is that *a client's aptitude for topic initiation, maintenance, change and termination be observed, with particular reference to how these are achieved rather than whether they occur or not.*

Non-linguistic communicative behaviour

In face to face communicative interactions verbal communication is normally accompanied by various forms of body language. These include facial expressions and eye contact, a certain amount of gesticulation by the hands, and body postures as well as distance from one's interlocutors. Another set of behaviours which are not strictly verbal, although involving the vocal apparatus, is the set of paralinguistic behaviours which also may have communicative functions. Among these are such prosodic features as volume, tone of voice, extra-emphatic stressing, exaggerated emphatic intonation and speed of delivery. In natural, neutral conversations all these go unnoticed. The moment they are noticeable they either function as additional communicative devices or as some form of disorder. It is impossible to state categorically to what degree their presence is 'normal'. The reason for this is that many of them are not measurable behaviours, and even if they were the appropriate measures are likely to be different for different individuals. Thus, whereas a certain amount of eye contact is desirable, especially at the beginning and end of a speaker's turn, constant exaggerated eye fixation can be threatening, defiant or abnormal, making the conversational partner uncomfortable. Too little of it can be equally disturbing. Similarly, too little body distance can be regarded either as overconfident or as threatening, but equally too great a distance is just as perturbing. The same applies to the paralinguistic features. Monotone delivery can signal boredom, depression, mockery or could be construed as a disorder, just as exaggerated intonation contours may convey doubt, surprise, anger or could be a sign of disorder. Many of the existing communication profiles devote a great deal of attention to scoring clients on these non-verbal components of communication. Our suggestion is that *the non-linguistic and paralinguistic components of communication should be observed, but only to the extent that they are relevant to the overall picture regarding a client's communicative abilities.*

Presupposed knowledge

Presupposed knowledge is the kind of knowledge whose application is not specifically restricted to communication but without which communication is not possible. This involves knowledge about the world, assumptions and perceptions about the communicative environment, ability to make inferences and knowledge of the language.

A person's encyclopaedic knowledge, in other words what she or he knows about the world in general, is apt to influence the type and range of topics she or he is able to communicate about. Although this is self-evident, it is worth bearing in mind when creating communicative settings for any client, and particularly important with adults with learning disabilities. This client group deserves special attention because of the sometimes restricted nature of their world knowledge. It is perfectly possible that an individual does not know much about the transport system but is exceptionally well informed about, say, music or football. Therefore it is essential that, in any communication assessment, the client's special expertise or lack of it be taken into consideration.

As has been pointed out several times throughout this discussion, the nature of the communicative environment is of paramount significance in what counts as appropriate choice of topic, and appropriate choice of modalities to express the various communicative functions. These include requests or orders, for example, the amount of information necessary, the style of communication to be adopted and the way conversational devices are employed. Therefore it is essential that participants in a conversation have similar perceptions about the place, setting and purpose of the communicative event. It is also essential that they have the appropriate assumptions about each other's knowledge of the world, about each other's aspirations, sensitivities and needs. Failure on this can lead to unacceptable violations of the principle of relevance. Either too much or too little information is provided, or the partner is either unable to follow the speaker or finds the exchange insulting. At the extreme, complete breakdown of communication may result. In our view neither encyclopaedic knowledge nor assumptions and perceptions about the communicative environment lend themselves to exhaustive testing, important as it is to ascertain them. Therefore we suggest that *a client's general knowledge about the world and his or her perception of the communicative context and the communicative partners should be observed as a function of his or her communicative range and style.*

In view of what we have said about direct and indirect formulation of messages, and the many other features of a communicative situation, all of which can give rise to additional implications beyond the literal meaning of utterances, it is normally expected that speakers and hearers are capable of making inferences. There are two kinds of inference: logical entailments and pragmatic inferences. Logical entailments are those which are directly attributable to the linguistic content of an utterance. These are guaranteed by virtue of the words used and their meanings. Thus the word 'mother' logically entails the concept 'female'; the word 'rose' logically entails the concept 'flower'; the word 'run' in its literal meaning logically entails the concept of changing location. Thus the sentence: 'I saw your mother five minutes ago but I have not seen any women for the last 24 hours' is logically non-sensical. Understanding the logical connection between two expressions in this sense is an important part of both making discourse cohesive and perceiving it as such.

Pragmatic inferences, by contrast, are not guaranteed by the meanings of words used alone. They need to be supplemented by world knowledge, knowledge of conversational partners and shared assumptions about the communicative environment. So, a speaker's assertion that he or she does not like alcoholic drinks can give rise to a host of inferences. The listener would be behaving inappropriately by then offering beer, for example. But the listener may also infer that the speaker is a bore, or alternatively, a virtuous person or even a health freak, none of which is logically implied by the original assertion. Examples 2, 3 and 4 at the beginning of this chapter can only work if the right pragmatic inferences are drawn. Inference making is essential in normal everyday conversation. It is because of this property of communication that it has been defined by many authors as mutual 'negotiation' of meaning. The ability to both recognise logical entailments and make pragmatic inferences can be tested, and because of the all-prevalent nature of these we suggest that *a client's ability to recognise logical entailments and to make pragmatic inferences may need to be assessed.*

The last type of presupposed knowledge is the knowledge of language. In order to discuss what is involved we need to outline the linguistic framework.

The Linguistic Framework

Many readers are, no doubt, familiar with a number of different linguistic descriptions. The framework we are suggesting here is not necessarily superior to other models of language; we prefer it because it focuses on meaning and the ways in which language encodes meaning. It is this focus which enables us to create a link between linguistic structures and pragmatics, for the purposes of assessing communicative abilities. What follows is no more than an outline of those features of language which we suggest may need to be investigated, but we hope that enough explanation and exemplification will have been provided to enable even the novice to linguistics to make some use of it.

Language is essentially a code system in which meanings are encoded in arbitrary but systematic ways. The simplest meaningful codes are lexical items (or 'words', see below). The number of lexical items in a language is not only finite but rather limited compared to the range of meanings which need to be encoded. Therefore, lexical items are combined into such syntactic structures as phrases and clauses or sentences. One can go beyond clauses, as text linguists do, but for our purposes the clause is going to be the maximal construct. So, we say that the codes of language are the lexical items, phrases and clauses that correspond to concepts. Concepts are mental representations of the world. Virtually every concept that can be encoded by a lexical item can also be encoded by more complex structures such as phrases and clauses, but it is not the case the other way round. For example, take the concept JEALOUSY, for which there exists the lexical item 'jealousy'. The same concept is referred to in the *Shorter Oxford English Dictionary's* definition formulated as a phrase: 'the state of mind arising from the suspicion, apprehension or knowledge of rivalry'. Similarly, the word 'anger' can be expressed by a phrase, such as 'make someone angry'. Note, however, that the expression 'make someone laugh' cannot be expressed by a single lexical item.

For both theoretical and empirical reasons language is best regarded as being composed of a number of subsystems. These are:

1. The lexicon, which is the list of all lexical items (these can be words, morphemes and idioms) together with a specification of those phonological, morphological, syntactic and semantic properties which are not predictable by the rules and principles of any of the other subsystems.
2. Morphology, which is the system relating to the internal structure of words and to the principles of word formation.
3. Syntax, which is the linear and hierarchical organisation of phrases up to the level of clause (henceforward abbreviated as S).
4. Semantics, which is the meaning structure of words, phrases and Ss, and the meaning relations between words, phrases and Ss.
5. Phonology, which is the the sound system of language.

Each subsystem can be described as an autonomous component of language with its own set of rules and principles. For the purposes of communication assessments, what is of more interest is the way they interact with each other at the different levels of sentence structure. We shall accordingly discuss the semantic, syntactic and morphological features, as appropriate, at the level of single word, phrase structure and sentence structure. We will say nothing about phonology, as this is the aspect of language that is most familiar to most speech and language therapists, and as there exist some very useful assessment methods for this subsystem. For a detailed list and brief description of each assessment the reader is referred to Kersner's *Tests of Voice, Speech and Language* (Kersner, 1992).

Single word level – the lexicon

The term 'word' is problematic for linguistic theories because of the impossibility of finding a valid and satisfactory definition for it, and so linguists prefer to use the term 'lexical item'. Having established what a lexical item is, we shall continue to use the term 'word' informally, for the sake of ease of reading. The basic building blocks of all expressions are lexical items. These can correspond to units which we know informally as 'words'. They can correspond to meaningful units out of which words can be formed, otherwise known as 'morphemes', for example affixes, such as 'un' in the word 'unhappy'. They can correspond to those frozen expressions, otherwise known as 'idioms', which are largely unchangeable in different contexts and whose meaning is divorced from the meaning of their component words, e.g. 'to beat about the bush'. Lexical items can be characterised by their phonological, semantic and syntactic properties.

Semantic properties of lexical items

There are several ways in which the semantic properties, or meanings, of lexical items can be characterised. Words in themselves are not meaningful: it is only in context that they acquire meaning. One such context is the world surrounding us. Accordingly, words acquire meaning through their relationship with various entities and phenomena in the world. This type of meaning is referred to as referential meaning, where words can be regarded as names or labels. Another way the meaning of words can be thought of is as a correspondence relationship with the concepts they encode. The third way has to do with the kinds of relations that exist between lexical items.

The referential meaning of words is purely conventional and, of course, more than one word can refer to the same object, e.g. 'Mozart' , 'Viennese composer', 'child genius', etc. Some words have no referential meaning, for example 'if', 'but' , 'then' etc.

The conceptual approach to meaning has been developed by Jackendoff (1983), according to whom it is possible to isolate a very limited number of basic conceptual categories from which all others derive. One may argue about the choice of these categories but the ones we think are most relevant are listed in the following table, using Jackendoff's terminology (Jackendoff, 1983):

Category	Description	Examples
THING	Physical entities	Dog, gun, daughter, map, iron, paint
EVENT	Actions, happenings (physical or mental)	Go, fall, lecture, iron, paint, explode, occur
STATE	Physical, mental or emotional states	Sleep, broken, confused, love, sick
CAUSE	Causation of event or state	Upset (i.e. cause to become upset), send (i.e. cause something to go), anger (i.e. cause to become angry)
PLACE	Location, direction, path	In, to, from, along, via
TIME	Temporal expressions	Now, then, until, since
POSSESSION	Possession	My, your, of, mother's
PROPERTY	Qualities, characteristics	Green, warm, clever, genius, fool
QUANTITY	Quantity	Two, many, several, some

Each of these can be further subdivided into subcategories, for example in the case of THING, this can be ANIMATE THING or INANIMATE THING. If ANIMATE THING, it can be HUMAN or NON-HUMAN. The subclassification can go on in principle until one arrives at an individual object. For the purposes of analysis it is sometimes sufficient to stop at the top level, whereas on other occasions quite detailed subclassification may be necessary. EVENTS can also be subclassified according to whether action or a happening is involved. ACTIONS can further be subclassified according to whether or not change of place is involved. Although differently formulated and differently organised, these conceptual subclasses are not very different from the types of semantic field listed in Crystal (1982).

Some of these concepts are simple and others complex, in that they necessarily involve some other concept. So, as a rule, THING concepts are simple, whereas almost all EVENT concepts involve at least another concept, usually at least a THING. Take the word 'sleep'. This necessarily involves someone, i.e. a THING, whereas the word 'love' necessarily involves two other concepts, i.e. two THINGS, one who loves and one who is loved. Those additional concepts which are necessarily implied by a word's meaning are called its 'arguments'. We can thus talk about the meaning structure, or semantic structure, of words, in terms of the type of concept they correspond to and the number of arguments they take.

The relationships that hold between the lexical items of the language can be expressed by the familiar sense relations which themselves involve logical implications. These include:

1. Synonymy, where two words have identical meaning, e.g. 'dress' and 'frock'.
2. The various oppositions:
   (a) binary, e.g. 'single' and 'married';
   (b) gradable, e.g. 'tall' and 'short';
   (c) converse, e.g. 'buy' and 'sell';
   (d) multiple, e.g. 'rose', 'tulip', 'violet' and all the other flowers.
3. Inclusion, where the meaning of one word is included in the other, e.g. 'car' and 'vehicle'.

Syntactic properties of words

On the basis of their distribution words belong to various syntactic categories. Distribution is the set of sentence positions in which a word can occur. The most important syntactic categories are the following:

Noun (N)	e.g. table, shop, Jeremy, arrival, understanding as in 'my table/shop/Jeremy/arrival/understanding'
Verb (V)	e.g walk, cook, heal, suffer, like, understand as in 'he walked/cooked/healed/suffered/liked/understood'
Preposition (P)	e.g. with, in, about, since, after, like as in 'with/in/about/since/after/like my arrrival'
Adjective (A)	e.g. slim, pretty, elegant, proud, understanding as in 'She was slim/pretty/elegant/proud/understanding'
Adverb (Adv)	e.g. prettily, elegantly, proudly, understandingly as in 'She walked prettily/elegantly/proudly'
Determiner (Det)	e.g. the, a, this, my, your, his, her as in 'the/a/this/my/your/his or her table'
Quantifier (Q)	e.g. some, all, no, more as in 'some/all/no/more tables'
Auxiliary (Aux)	e.g. can, shall, have, be as in 'he can/shall walk'; 'have walked'; 'is walking'

Notice that not every single word one comes across in a text will fit into the above categories. For practical purposes this does not matter. Rather than force them into a category we can just cite such a word when we come across it. For example 'to' as in 'to kill' is not a member of any category.

The examples above illustrate that there is not a one to one correspondence between the meaning categories and the syntactic categories. So, for example, an N can represent the following meaning categories:

THING – cat, man, table
EVENT – walk, talk, concert
STATE – love, sleep, health

PLACE – home, inside
PROPERTY – genius, fool, beauty
QUANTITY – loads, heaps etc..

Another syntactic property of words is that they determine which of their arguments need to be expressed and which are optional when used in a sentence context. They also determine what syntactic category their arguments may be expressed by. This property is called, in modern usage the 'subcategorisation property' of words. The notion is familiar in traditional grammar as well. One used to say a word 'takes' such and such a complement. To exemplify: take the words 'arrive', 'come' and 'reach', in the following sentences:

1. Tim arrived at Victoria Station.
2. Tim came to Victoria Station.
3. Tim reached Victoria Station.

In Sentences 1 and 2 the verbs 'arrive' and 'come' take prepositional complements, in fact involving two different prepositions. They are not interchangeable. It would be incorrect to say 'Tim arrived to Victoria Station' or 'Tim came at Victoria Station'. There is no logical reason for the choice of a particular preposition: it is the idiosyncratic property of these verbs that they select one or the other. In the case of 'reach' the verb takes a noun complement. It would be wrong to replace this by either of the prepositional complements. Furthermore, although all three verbs have some place designation necessarily implied in their meaning – in other words they all have this concept as one of their arguments – only in the case of 'reach' is it obligatory to give it overt expression. 'Tim arrived' and 'Tim came' are both acceptable English sentences, whereas 'Tim reached' is not. This is another instance where although there is a connection between the meaning of the words and the syntax associated with them, there is no one to one correspondence.

Phrase level

Although the meaning of words can be quite complex, in that several concepts can be incorporated, there is a limit to the number of concepts that can be expressed by single words. Therefore, words need to be combined into more complex syntactic structures called sentences. However , these are not structured directly from words; there are various layers of phrases that serve as building blocks which ultimately form the sentence. Phrases minimally consist of a 'head' which is the same syntactic category as the phrase itself. So noun phrases (NPs) have N, verb phrases (VPs) have V, adjectival phrases (APs) have A, prepositional phrases (PP)s have P, adverbial phrases (AdvPs) and quantifier phrases (QP) have Q as their heads. From the point of view of

meaning it is this head that the constituent 'is about'. The subcategorisation of the head determines what 'complements' can follow it in a
sentence. From a semantic point of view the complements are the arguments associated with the concept that the head corresponds to. Apart
from the head and the complements, phrases may also contain other
modifiers, sometimes referred to as 'restrictive modifiers'. The head
and its arguments, if these are expressed, can function as a 'referring
expression', referring to a type of EVENT or STATE or THING etc. The
role of the restrictive modifiers is to limit or restrict the range of potential referents of the referring expression. For example, in the sentence:
'Tim arrived at Victoria Station the other day' there is a VP:

arrived	*at Victoria Station*	*the other day*
Head	Complement	
EVENT	Argument	Restrictive modifier
	(PLACE)	

'Arrive' is a word that corresponds to an EVENT concept. As its meaning
involves movement from one place to another, some place designation
is necessarily implied. In this sentence the PP: 'at Victoria Station'
fulfils this requirement and is, therefore, the argument of the head. The
time of arrival is not necessarily implied, but it serves to restrict the reference to that 'arrival at Victoria Station' which happened 'the other
day'.

The PP: 'at Victoria Station' can be analysed in a similar way:

at	*Victoria Station*
Head	Complement
PLACE	Argument
	(THING)

In this expression there is no restrictive modifier. The NP: 'the other
day' is also analysable in the same way:

the	*other*	*day*
		Head
Restrictive		TIME
modifiers		

In this expression there are no arguments. The syntactic category of
the arguments is, as discussed earlier, determined in an idiosyncratic
way by the subcategorisation properties of the head. The syntactic category of the modifiers, on the other hand, is determined by the syntactic
category of the head. So, for example, nouns can be modified by a

preceding AP, a QP and/or a determiner (Det), and by a following PP or relative clause, e.g.

the	little	prince	in the story	who loved a fox
		Head		
Det	AP	N	PP	Relative clause

Verbs can be modified by a following NP, PP, AdvP and by an infinitive VP, as in:

(He) danced	most elegantly	last night	at the party	to impress Jane
Head				
V	AdvP	NP	PP	inf. VP

Sentence level

Phrases combine to form clauses or sentences. We shall use the convention marking clauses with 'S', which stands for both clauses and sentences. What makes an S different from a phrase is that it does not have a head as such. There are some linguists who claim that clauses are nothing more than a special case of VPs. According to these theoreticians, clauses have Vs as their heads and what makes them special is that, instead of having all the complements, or arguments following the head, one of them will precede it. This is termed the 'external argument' and can also be referred to as the 'subject' of the sentence. Irrespective of whether we want to regard Ss as special VPs or not, it is true that the V has a major role. It is the verb's meaning that determines what concept or combination of concepts the whole S corresponds to. For example the S: 'Kathie drove the car through the forest' is about an EVENT whose main exponent is the verb 'drive' and the rest of S is its arguments: the THING (+ human) who did the driving, the THING (-human) that she drove and the PLACE (path) where she drove. The S: 'Kathie suffers from migraines' is about a STATE, represented by the verb 'suffer' and again, the other constituents are its arguments: 'Kathie', a THING (+human) and 'migraines', a STATE.

Verbs also play an important role in that they assign different 'semantic roles' to their arguments in an S. These semantic roles, also referred to as 'thematic roles' are taken from Jackendoff (1972). He suggested that they might overcome the problems of separating the syntactic and semantic properties of the grammatical functions 'subject' and 'object'. Traditionally, subject was often defined in notional terms, as the 'doer' or 'agent', and object as the ' 'patient' or 'the thing affected'. Both subject and object are useful and valid concepts from the point of view of the syntactic organisation of Ss, but they can both take on a variety of semantic or thematic roles, just as the other verb complements can.

To summarise, the following thematic roles have been proposed (in the following examples the expressions which are assigned the thematic role under discussion will be italicised):

1. *Agent:* the instigator of some action. It is often assumed in the linguistic literature that agenthood involves wilful action and therefore only human entities are candidates for this role. One can take a more flexible attitude and include animals as well as natural forces. If there is an agent in a sentence, then normally this role is represented by the subject NP, e.g.

   The enemy destroyed the capital.

   The bull destroyed the china shop.

   The storm destroyed the forest.

2. *Theme*: the entity whose position or whose movement the verb asserts, e.g.

   There are *some tiles* in the back garden.

   The tiles have fallen off the roof.

   The wind blew *the tiles* off the roof.

   If the entity whose movement the verb asserts is animate there could be ambiguity as to whether to assign it the thematic role of agent or theme. For example in 'The boy ran across the street' one could argue that 'the boy' is both the instigator and the entity whose movement the verb asserts. In this case it is acceptable to assign both roles, although the meaning of the verb seems to focus more on an Agent interpretation. In the sentence 'The boy floated on the water', however, the meaning of the verb focuses more on the theme interpretation than on the agent interpretation. The concept of theme can be extended in some more abstract domains, such as time, or some scale of measurement or possession or identity.

   e.g. Time:

   The football match took place at 5 p.m.

   We postponed *the football match* till next weekend.

   Scale of measurement:

   We kept *the distance* at 2 feet.

   The temperature increased to its highest level.

   Possession:

   The guitar belongs to my son.

   He lost *his briefcase*.

   Bill gave me *his gold watch*.

   Identity:

   He remained a bachelor.

   That pretty girl turned into an old witch.

3. *Patient:* the entity 'affected' by some action carried out by the agent, if the verb of the S does not involve static position change of location, e.g.

   The cook spoilt *the broth.*

   The teacher scolded *the boys.*

   It is important to note that some of the literature does not distinguish between patient and theme but uses theme to refer to both.

4. *Experiencer:* the entity experiencing some physical, mental or psychological state, e.g.

   Kathie suffers from migraines.

   My mother remembers all my misdeeds.

   Some people hate linguistics.

5. *Stimulus:* the entity that is the cause of the above states, e.g. in the above sentences 'from migraines', 'all my misdeeds' and 'linguistics' are all assigned the role of stimulus.

6. *Location:* place where something is situated or takes place, e.g.

   John keeps the books *on the shelf.*

   The garden was swarming with bees.

7. *Goal:* the place towards which movement takes place, or the end point of movement, e.g.

   John passed the *book to Mary.*

   Bill gave *me* his gold watch.

   The room filled with smoke..

8. *Source:* the place from which movement takes place, e.g.

   Mary came *from the moon.*

   My uncle left me a fortune.

   The glass emptied in seconds.

Another important set of meaning characteristics of sentences, also largely expressed within the VP, are tense, aspect and mood. As speech and language therapists are perhaps more familiar with these concepts than with the foregoing, we shall not go into a very detailed account of these. Essentially, tense, expressed by past and present tense morphemes, relates to the time of an event or state relative to the time of an utterance. However, there is no one to one correspondence between tense as a grammatical marker and time as a semantic concept. Thus the present tense can refer to timeless states of affairs, as in 'John smokes cigars', 'The earth goes round the sun in approximately 24 hours'. It can also refer to future events, e.g. 'I start working next week'. It can even refer to past events in the so-called narrative past, e.g. 'I was sitting on the bus minding my own business when this man comes up to me and tells me to move over.' Similarly, the past tense form of a verb does not necessarily refer to past time. For example, in the sentence: 'I was wondering if you could do me a favour', 'was' and 'could' are both past tense forms but refer to present time.

The progressive and perfect aspects refer roughly to a distinction between whether an event or state is being regarded as ongoing or as completed. Syntactically they are expressed by the auxiliaries 'be' and 'have', respectively, with the appropriate morphological form of the following verb. So, for example, 'I am reading the papers' refers to some ongoing event, whereas 'I have read the papers' implies that I have finished reading.

Mood, again roughly, refers to the speaker's attitude to some event or state, or whether it is possible, or necessary in the world as it stands. Mood is expressed by the so-called 'modal auxiliaries' : can, may, must, shall and will. Tense, aspect and mood can interact to express still more dimensions of events and states.

For a very detailed account of these the reader is referred to Palmer (1965), Leech (1971) or Huddleston (1984).

Tense, aspect and mood are part of the pragmatic component of language. They only play a part in sentence meaning when sentences are embedded in context.

It is possible to summarise the type of syntactic and semantic features which are relevant at each level of S structure, bearing in mind that although they are related the correspondence is not one to one (Table 8.1).

Table 8.1 Syntactic and related semantic categories at word, phrase and sentence level.

	Syntactic	*Semantic*
Word level	Syntactic categories Subcategorisation properties	Semantic categories Argument structure
Phrase level	Head Complements Other constituents	Main concept Arguments Restrictive modifiers
Sentence level	Grammatical functions and other complements Tense Auxiliaries	Thematic roles Time Aspect and mood

It is possible that problems occur on any one level, in either the syntactic or the semantic subsystem. This may have serious adverse implications for communicative effectiveness. Therefore we suggest that *clients' linguistic abilities on all levels and subsystems may need to be assessed.*

Guidelines for Communication Assessment

Having established what we may need to assess, the next question is how one can bring together all the various threads of this very complex phenomenon called communication. We are going to attempt to find answers for the following questions:

1. What are the purposes of any one particular assessment?
2. How do we elicit data for the assessment?
3. How do we analyse these data?
4. How do we evaluate the results of our analysis?
5. How can we use the results for intervention or management purposes?

The purposes of assessment

We discussed in some detail in Chapter 2 the desirability of assessing communicative abilities in general. In the case of adults with learning disabilities the purposes of assessment fall into two main categories:

1. Rehabilitation/management, with the ultimate aim of enabling the client to lead a more independent life.
2. Research.

We are still some way away from fully understanding learning disorders in general and the interplay between these and communication skills in particular. The two purposes may require different depth and scope of assessment. Within the first category there are also at least two different considerations: the assessment can be undertaken either with the aim of trying to improve the communication skills of the clients, or in order to influence the environment in which the client lives, to maximise the use of existing abilities.

How do we elicit data?

Whatever the purpose of assessment, the first practical step is the collection of data. Different authors specify different criteria for what type of data is most useful and informative. This question is as relevant for the evaluation of communication in adults with learning disabilities as it is in any other client group. There is considerable literature on this topic in the field of second language learning. The points at issue are: what constitutes a representative sample of behaviour? How much data are necessary? Is the assessment of each individual component of communication a worthwhile undertaking? To quote Oller and Khan (1981, p. 28): 'Should we never try to measure one and only one point of one and only one component of one and only one aspect of one and only one skill? The answer seems to be yes, we should never try that. Why? Simply because any such attempt to isolate bits and pieces of language destroys the fabric of language.' They go on, however: 'On the other hand, there are circumstances where it may be wise to focus on particular elements of language in context.... It can be done with integrative testing techniques where distinctive features, phonemes, morphemes, lexical items, syntactic patterns, pragmatic functions, notions, speech acts, illocutionary, perlocutionary and whatever other forces and elements interact to constitute discourse.' This is the spirit in which we are making our recommendations.

In collecting data a number of considerations need to be borne in mind. First and foremost is the fact that in any one communicative situation the client whom we assess is both speaker and hearer. Most communication profiles concentrate on the speaker's role and pay relatively little attention to the hearer's role. A second consideration is the 'naturalness' of the data. There are disparate views as to whether naturally occurring spontaneous data or data elicited in strictly controlled, test-like contexts are the more revealing (Dormandy and van der Gaag, 1989). Some profiles, for example CASP (van der Gaag, 1988), compromise by including both methods. We would suggest that both methods have merits as well as drawbacks. The obvious advantage of the spontaneous speech sample is that it is the most natural; the greatest disadvantage is that it is more or less out of the control of the assessor. Frequently, the assessor will compromise by creating a question/answer 'interview' type of situation. The advantage of language elicited under strictly controlled circumstances is that the assessor knows at least what the target is, and is therefore in a better position to form an accurate picture. In reality, some degree of compromise is necessary in all assessments of communication. Naturalness may need to be bought at the expense of control, or vice versa. Besides, there are techniques which fall between the two extremes and contain both elements to a greater or lesser degree. Again, we can learn from the literature on second language testing, where research in this field is well advanced. A helpful classification of elicited data would be as follows:

1. Communicative discourse
2. Pseudocommunicative discourse
3. Connected discourse
4 Controlled responses

Communicative discourse

This is the prototypical conversation. It often involves open-ended question/answer components or a more fixed version, such as asking for specific information, e.g. 'what's your name?', 'where do you live' and so on. It is also possible and useful to include some statement/ response component, where the assessor makes the kind of statement that normally invites a response, e.g something like: 'I'm sorry you had to wait so long'/'That's quite all right'. Another technique is to introduce ambiguities, unclear cues or even faulty information to provoke a self-initiated response from the client. For example, 'I'm sorry, did you say that you lived at...?' It is a particularly useful way to prompt clients to ask questions, for example.

Pseudocommunicative discourse

It clearly is not practical to wait for all topics and all contexts to emerge spontaneously. Therefore, data samples can be generated by techniques that give rise to almost natural conversational exchanges at the same time as giving the assessor some degree of control. One such technique is role play. Another, perhaps more natural one is the messenger role, where the client is asked to convey some information or direct some question or request to a third party, who could be a friend, a relative or a helper, who could send messages back.

Connected discourse

As a rule, conversational turns tend to be rather short. If the therapist wishes to evaluate a client's ability to maintain a longer stretch of continuous and cohesive speech there are a number of tasks that could elicit this. Such tasks include asking the client to tell or retell a story, give a report about some recent event, describe a typical day or a specific day in his or her life, explain how to do something or describe what a place or an object looks like. It is possible to vary both the level of difficulty and the degree of control.

Controlled responses

The prototypical method to elicit the most controlled responses is through tests. Because they are the least natural, their use should be restricted to investigating very specific aspects of language and communication, for example where the therapist suspects either that these are responsible for difficulties in communication or that their availability to the client can be utilised in forming communication strategies.

Almost all parameters of communication discussed earlier in the chapter can be tested. Care must be taken when designing a test, that the topic chosen is appropriate for an individual client; that tasks associated with speaker and those associated with hearer are kept separate: for example, if a client's comprehension or perception of some communication parameter is being tested, the output requirements should be kept to a minimum, if not to zero, by tasks that require no verbal output but where the response can be communicated by pointing, pressing buttons, nodding etc.; and that failure on one task can be unambiguously ascribed to one factor and that this is indeed what is being tested. For example, in a vocabulary test, failure on any one item should not be accountable for by phonological output problems.

How do we analyse the data?

Rather than using checklists as a basis for analysis, we suggest that therapists bear in mind all components of communication and include the type of questions outlined above in the discussion of the parameters of communication. We shall introduce two methods of analysis based on the pragmatic and linguistic framework discussed earlier in the chapter: a macro analysis and a microanalysis.

Macro level analysis

This, in our opinion, is adequate for arriving at an overall picture of a client's communicative abilities. It involves investigating the following: the range of contexts; the range of topics; the range of communicative purposes, say, speech acts; an observation of the client's non-linguistic and paralinguistic behaviour, from the point of view of whether these are appropriate, inappropriate, and whether they can be utilised to overcome shortcomings in other areas; the appropriateness of the client's responses in terms of, say, adjacency pairs and the principle of relevance.

In addition to these, the verbal component of communication can be assessed from the point of view of the range of semantic categories, and their corresponding lexical realisation, both in terms of choice of lexical item and syntactic category of the item, and the range of semantic (or thematic) roles, meanings expressed by restrictive modifiers and their corresponding syntactic, i.e. phrasal and clausal, realisation as well as aspectual and modal meaning, together with their syntactic exponents.

The first step in analysing the data is to ask: does the client use/understand words of different semantic types and does he or she express/understand them through the appropriate syntactic categories? The tables below give the correlations between meaning types and their syntactic realisations: in Table 8.2, for example, at the single word level.

The question to ask is: Does the client use and understand these word types in a variety of contexts?

The next question is: does the client form appropriate phrases and sentences from words to express the arguments and restrictive modifiers appropriately, and does she or he understand them? Table 8.3

Table 8.2 Semantic–pragmatic categories and related syntactic categories at single word level

Semantic/Pragmatic	Syntactic
Social terms	
e.g. *hello, thanks*	
proper vs. common terms for THINGS	N
e.g. proper: *Fido, Jack*	
common: *table, clock, horse, woman*	
EVENT terms:	
ACTION (– change of location)	V, N, A
e.g. V: *drink, play, saw*	
N: *party, performance, trip*	
A: *naughty, silly, abusive*	
ACTION (+ change of location)	V, N
e.g. V: *go, fly, travel*	
N: *flight, journey, drive*	
STATE terms:	V, N, A, P
e.g. V: *sleep, love, enjoy*	
N: *sleep, love, enjoyment*	
A: *sleepy, sick, happy*	
P: *up, down, off*	
CAUSE + ACTION:	V, N
e.g. V: *push, put, send*	
N: *push, dismissal, throw*	
CAUSE + STATE	V, N
e.g. V: *annoy, shorten, spoil*	
N: *destruction, rejection*	
PROPERTY terms	A, N, V
e.g. A: *tall, green, greedy*	
N: *height, colour, greediness*	
V: *drink, stutter, steal*	
(Note: V only works if these words are used to characterise a THING)	
PLACE terms	P, N
e.g. P: *here, at, inside*	
N: *home*	
POSSESSION terms	P, Det, Ns, Pronouns
e.g. P: *of*	
Det: *my, your, our*	
N's: *boy's, Jenny's, mother's*	
Pronoun: *mine, yours, ours*	
TEMPORAL terms	P, N, Aux, Suffixes
e.g. P: *at, after, before*	
N: *time, minute, year*	
Aux: *had, used to, will*	
Suffixes: *-s, ed* or irregular past	
QUANTITY terms	Numbers, Q, plural
e.g. Numbers: *1, 25, 156*	
Q: *many, few, all*	
Plural: *s* or irregular forms	
Deictic terms	Det, Pronoun, P
e.g. Det: *this, that*	
Pronoun: *this, that*	
P: *here, there*	

shows semantic–pragmatic categories and their related phrase structure at the sentence level.

Note that this is not a complete account of the grammar of English, but a selection of the most widely used meanings and their syntactic expressions; some of the syntactic expressions sound more contrived than others; there is no requirement that all of the possibilities should be utilised by any speaker on any one occasion.

An analysis of this kind has the advantage that not every single utterance of a client needs to be considered, therefore it is less time-con-

---

Table 8.3 Semantic–pragmatic categories and their related phrase structure at the sentence level

Semantic/Pragmatic	Syntactic
Thematic roles:	
Agent/action	NP, VP
e.g. *Johnny is eating.*	
Agent/action/theme	NP, V, NP
	NP, V, PP
e.g. *Johnny is pushing his friends.*	
The ball was thrown by Johnny.	
Agent/action/theme/goal	
or source	NP, V, NP, PP
e.g. Agent/action/theme goal:	
Johnny poured the wine into the glass.	
Johnny filled the glass with water.	
e.g. Agent/action/theme/source:	
Johnny took the money from the box.	
Johnny robbed the bank of all their cash	

(Note that the linear order of the thematic roles is not necessarily the same as that of the syntactic phrasal categories.)

Theme/action	NP, V
e.g. *Johnny is leaving.*	
Theme/action or state/location	
(or goal or source)	NP, V, PP
e.g. Theme/action or state/location:	
Johnny was standing in the corner	
Theme/action/goal:	
Johnny fell into the pond.	
The pond filled up with water.	
Theme/action/source:	
Johnny fell from the tree.	
The crowd disappeared from the square.	
The square was cleared of people.	

All the above can be extended to time, possession and identity, as explained under semantic roles.

Theme/property	NP, V, AP
e.g. *Johnny is skilled.*	or NP, V, NP
e.g. *Johnny is a fool.*	or NP, V
e.g. *Johnny steals.*	

suming than a full analysis. Where linguistic errors occur or the usage is inappropriate, this can be noted against the type of meaning or type of syntactic structure involved. Clinicians only need to scan through the data, particularly if they have a suspicion that some categories are 'missing' from a client's repertory or are expressed by the inappropriate form. Then it is useful to see, by comparison, with which categories, at which level, in what linguistic or non-linguistic context the client has no problems. This in turn can be utilised when deciding on intervention goals.

Table 8.3 *(contd)*

Semantic/Pragmatic	Syntactic
Experiencer/state/stimulus	NP, V, NP
e.g. *Johnny likes ice cream*	
	or NP, V, PP
e.g. *Johnny suffers from headaches.*	
Restrictive modifiers:	
Time	PP, NP
e.g. PP: *at noon, after dinner*	
after they left the cinema	
NP: *last night; the other day*	
Place PP	
e.g. *in the garden, at the cinema*	
Cause PP	
e.g. for *some reason*	
because of you	
because he is not kind	
Manner	AdvP, PP
e.g. AdvP: *skilfully, very elegantly*	
PP: *in a clumsy manner*	
etc.	
Progressive/perfect aspect	Aux V+ suffix
e.g. Progressive: *is going*	
Perfect: *has eaten*	
Mood Modal aux	
e.g. *will, shall, may, must*	

In addition, other syntactic features involve the appropriate use of:

- Word order in statements and commands
- Word order in questions
- Negatives
- Subject/verb agreement
- Use of complex sentences.

Micro level analysis

This method of analysis is more appropriate for research, or if therapists feel that a full utterance by utterance analysis of a client's verbal
abilities in various communication contexts is called for. Again, the
choice of the particular pragmatic or linguistic model is not quite as
important as the adoption of the integrated approach. We suggest that
information relating to the context, main topic, participants and their
relationship can be stated, say at the top of the page. This would be followed by a five-column table, the five columns being headed :

1. Pragmatic information
2. Semantic roles and other meanings
3. Phrase structure
4. Semantic categories
5. Lexical items.

The information recorded in each column is:

1. Pragmatic information: purpose (in terms of speech act), whether
   the utterance represents a new turn or not, whether the utterance
   introduces a new topic or not, whether it contains some cohesive
   device or not, whether there are any overly lengthy pauses, any styl-
   istic remark that the therapist may wish to make, any disturbing or
   inappropriate non-linguistic or paralinguistic behaviour if it inter-
   feres, and whether the content of the utterance was relevant or not.
   This information could be coded as shown in the table below.
2. Semantic roles and other meanings: the types of information that
   are outlined earlier in the macro level method, e.g. agent/action/
   theme etc., listed after the question: 'Can the client form sentences?'
3. Phrase structure: the kind of phrasal analysis associated with semantic roles and other meanings of the macro level method.
4. Semantic categories: the type of concepts we discussed under the
   heading 'Linguistic framework'.
5. Lexical items: the actual words used together with the syntactic categories to which the words belong.

Any errors in syntax, any inappropriate meaning category or wrong
choice of word can be indicated by an asterisk against them.

What follows is a short excerpt from a conversation between a client
and staff member at a day centre for adults with learning disabilities:

Staff: You cooked your own breakfast, did you?
Client: Yeah.
Staff: What did you cook for breakfast?
Client: I cooked fried eggs.
Staff: And anything else?

Client: And bacon. Me mum cooks too. But she's on holiday now. I went to the seaside once.

The following table is an example of micro analysis:

CONTEXT: day centre, informal conversation
PARTICIPANTS: staff and client
TOPIC: cooking

Pragmatic information	Semantic roles and other meanings	Phrase structure	Semantic category	Lexical items
Inform Response, new turn	Ag/act/patient Past	NP, V, NP	THING ACT	I (N) cooked(V)
			THING	fried eggs (N)
Inform, response cohesive				and
	Patient	NP	THING	bacon (N)
Inform, self-init	Ag/act	NP, V	Poss	me (det)
			THING ACT	mum (N) cooks(V)
cohesive				too
Inform, self-init New topic	Theme/st/loc	NP, V, PP	THING STATE PLACE THING	she (N) 's in London (N)
	Time			now (P)
Inf. self-init *new topic	Ag/act/goal	NP, V, PP	THING ACT	I (N) go
	Time			-ed
			PLACE	to (P)
	Deictic			the (Det)
			THING	seaside (N)
	Time			once

How do we evaluate the results?

We have argued that the purpose of communication assessments in the clinical context is to establish the quality of a client's communicative abilities. Given the multifaceted nature of communication assessment procedures, their evaluation also needs to be multidimensional. There are three separate but related levels on which evaluation may need to be undertaken: the first we could call the behavioural level, which involves a careful analysis of the client's abilities regarding any one component of communication. The question to be asked is: are the behaviours, both linguistic and non-linguistic, appropriate? This level needs to be supplemented by the functional level, which examines how inappropriate behaviours may afftect communicative effectiveness, if at all, and whether existing abilities can be utillised to improve it.

The assessment methods outlined in this chapter are capable of providing answers to questions at both the behavioural and the functional level. The results of the assessment of the behavioural level are measurable and may even be scorable. The results of the functional level are not. They require qualitative evaluation, as discussed in Chapter 3.

The third level of evaluation requires a psycholinguistics-orientated approach. This locates both the problems and abilities within the communication processing mechanism. It may provide explanations as to the causes of specific problems and can provide ways of overcoming them. This approach is widely used with aphasic adults (Byng, 1988; Lesser, 1989) but still needs to be explored in relation to adults with learning disabilities.

Intervention based on the integrated model of communication assessment

As the model is first offered here we are not in a position to report on its efficacy from the point of view of intervention. It clearly awaits testing on large numbers of individuals. However, in line with the unquestionable principle that it is on the basis of assessment that goals of intervention or management can be determined, we suggest that the assessment will provide guidelines as to what these goals should be. Broadly, there are three types of goal that can be set:

1. Change the behaviour: in other words, either try to improve the linguistic and non-linguistic skills that make up communication, or teach the client to make use of available abilities, to compensate for problem areas. There is some literature in the area of second language teaching as to the kind of strategies people use to overcome problems, and how these can be utilised in teaching (Bialystok, 1990).
2. Change the environment: Chapters 6 and 7 of this book discussed some of the philosophies and the kinds of environment that are relevant for adults with learning disabilities. These philosophies go some way towards helping to create environments in which adults with learning difficulties are able to function and fulfil their potential. This is an essential prerequisite for effective communication. The kinds of change in the environments that we are considering here can be achieved by effecting changes in local attitudes to disability and improving clients' lives by giving them more choices and

more opportunities.

3. Teach the carers and others to accommodate to the client's behaviour by becoming more consciously sensitive to the different components of communication and their inhibiting or facilitating effects.

In keeping with the multidimensional theme of this book it is quite likely that aspects of more than one of these goals will apply for any one client.

Chapter 9
Research Directions

The Link between Evaluative Research and Accountability

This chapter discusses research issues as they relate to communication and adults with learning disabilities. One major concern is with the application of research methods in the clinical context. This is becoming increasingly important as health care professionals at all levels are being asked to give a more studied account of how they use resources. The chill winds of market forces blow strong (Griffiths, 1988; DOH, 1989). Donabedian's (1980) suggestion that 'our responsibility (as clinicians) is to provide the highest quality of care using the least amount of resources' echoes somewhat despairingly in the corridors of public service establishments around the country. The reason there is despair is partly because practitioners are being asked to undertake more and more 'measurement' with fewer and fewer resources, and partly because there is a more fundamental problem with defining 'highest quality of care'. What constitutes the highest quality of speech and language therapy for an adult with a learning disability? How can it be measured? The recent trend towards an acceptance of more functional outcomes does help to direct these questions to some extent. Kent (1989) observed that it is not enough to know that behavioural management produces behavioural change: 'We must know that it works for the overall benefit of the client in his or her social milieu. It must increase functional capacity to achieve (relevant) life goals' (p.7).

Much of the work outlined in previous chapters of this book is helping to achieve this goal. Therapists are increasingly functionally orientated, concerned not only with achievements in client–therapist interactions but with achievements in the wider social milieu – interactions with peers, family, carers, shopowners, publicans etc. The difficulties are not with the concept of achieving functional outcomes, but with knowing how to assess them accurately. Would a therapist know, for example, which type of intervention had a proven effectiveness with a certain type of communication difficulty?

There is a lack of information on the relative merits and demerits of different types of intervention. This has been observed across all areas of communication intervention. Tallal (1988) expressed her concerns in this sobering statement:

> 'The role of the interventionist can only be defined when theoretical issues regarding the nature of language, language disorders, and language change are better understood. This will require research investigating the assumptions under which clinicians currently operate; systematic, programmatic research is needed to address the major intervention assumptions and to generate principles for making informed clinical judgements' (p.253).

In the light of previous chapters, this seems a little gloomy. As McReynolds (1990) points out, research into the efficacy of different therapeutic approaches (we shall call it treatment efficacy for short) has an even shorter history than applied communication disorders research in general - only starting in earnest in the 1970s. McReynolds conducted an extensive survey of treatment efficacy research in the USA and was more optimistic than Tallal: she concluded that the field was showing signs of a growing interest and commitment to research.

As part of her review, McReynolds undertook a national survey of clinicians' attitudes to research (Kelly and McReynolds, 1988); 1000 questionnaires were sent to clinicians throughout the USA, 35% of whom responded. The survey asked whether they thought that naturalistic settings were an appropriate location for conducting clinical research; whether clinicians should be engaged in research; and whether they thought clinicians had the necessary research skills to undertake such studies. The results showed that clinicians were strongly in favour of research: 93% though that their interventions should be evaluated, and 95% said that, as clinicians, they should be involved in research. However, only 40% said that they thought they had the skills necessary to undertake such work; the remainder said that they were 'inadequately prepared' at college for designing and conducting research. This finding is in line with ASHA's (1980) observation that less than 1% of its members give research as their 'primary employment activity'. Had such a survey been carried out in the UK, there would probably have been very similar findings.

In their conclusions, Kelly and McReynolds stressed that, until more clinicians became actively engaged in research, there would be a lack of valuable treatment efficacy studies. More studies would result in more efficient treatment delivery systems. This statement is very much in line with the prevailing ideas and observations in this book. As we have seen in earlier chapters, there is still very little proven efficacy in the field of speech and language therapy for people with learning disabilities, still less a wealth of replicated studies.

The need for replication

Barlow et al. (1984), placed great emphasis on the need for those involved in clinical research to replicate each other's findings, regardless of what methodology they choose. It is only through replication that sound theories can emerge, and that interventions can become applicable to more individuals (Aylwin, 1988; Eastwood, 1988; Bench, 1989). Cronbach (1975) called this 'intensive local observation', a willingness to observe the successes and failures of a particular intervention, and to analyse the reasons for individual variations. In order to achieve this, clinicians must have a commitment to careful record keeping over a period of time. Ingham et al. (1990) stressed that, for efficacy studies to prove useful in the development of better interventions, replication of outcomes is crucial. They recommended a number of techniques, including the use of before and after measures with different clients who were participating in the same intervention. They advocated measuring communication skills in a variety of settings using a variety of measurement techniques, for example, video recordings, questionnaires for carers etc. They also recommended evaluating large numbers of clients in different locations working with a variety of therapists: a multicentre approach. As far as we are aware, no such studies are being undertaken in relation to the communication of adults with learning disabilities on a scale that would allow replication of the effects of different interventions. As we observed in Chapter 4, even the latest developments in communication assessments in the UK lack the research (as yet) to give reliable and valid data.

Chapter 3 discussed the importance of social validity for communication assessments. This is of equal importance in relation to intervention. Goldstein (1990) suggests that the 'social relevance' of a particular intervention is important as a measure of its efficacy. Are the goals of the intervention socially relevant?

Another complicating factor in the call to deliver the highest quality of care for the least amount of resource is that there remains some confusion in our understanding of the term 'treatment efficacy' itself. Olswang (1990) proposes three quite separate elements:

1. Treatment effectiveness, which refers to the validity of a particular treatment and asks 'Does the treatment work or not?'
2. Treatment efficiency, which examines the relative merits of one approach over another in a given context and asks 'Does therapy A work better than therapy B?'
3. Treatment effects, which is concerned with the influence of the therapy and asks 'In what ways has this therapy altered the client's behaviour?'

Olswang goes on to say that, traditionally, most treatment efficacy research has focused on the first two, but more recent trends favour the third. In the UK, the question of 'value for money' in health care has brought greater emphasis on treatment efficiency. Rosen and Proctor's (1981) discussion of therapeutic outcome provides some helpful guidance on how treatment effects might be measured. They distinguished between three types of treatment outcome:

1. Intermediate outcomes: for example, day to day recordings of therapy sessions, case notes on a client's progress;
2. Instrumental outcomes: how much therapy does it take to trigger a particular action or behaviour, for example, using a specific sound for the first time in conversation?
3. Ultimate outcomes: the outcomes that actually have social validity for the client, that is, they make a difference in everyday interactions.

Frattelli (1986) identified the utilisation of intermediate outcomes as one of speech and language therapy's strengths. Certainly, there is much in this book to support her observation. For example, most of the communication assessment techniques outlined in Chapter 4 make extensive use of intermediate outcomes, better known as goal planning and objective setting. These are one way of arriving at intermediate outcomes.

Frattelli asserts that the first stage in developing outcomes is to improve our record-keeping systems and to refine our use of task-orientated goals. We would suggest that speech and language therapists working with adults with learning disabilities are already working within this milieu. The principles of goal planning (Houts and Scott, 1975) are embedded firmly in our approaches to assessment and intervention, whether consciously or not. Identifying specific objectives, describing how these objectives might be achieved, who is to be involved and when progress is to be evaluated are all common knowledge now, if not common practice. In short, this area of communication intervention has the basis for developing a catalogue of its successes and failures: it has a methodology on line which contributes significantly to defining treatment outcomes.

But what about instrumental and ultimate outcomes? The difficulty, of course, is in determining exactly what and who is responsible for changes in a client's communication skills. Is it the intervention technique itself? Is it the therapeutic relationship? Is it an aspect of the environment? Is it the timing? This is where the path becomes less well defined and is most difficult to determine, given the problems of introducing randomised controlled trials and other controlled means of health services evaluation (see below).

The first stage in tackling such issues is to develop some way of measuring change over time, as discussed in an earlier chapter. The second stage is to develop the tools which can identify all the possible influences on those changes. Barlow et al. (1984) recommend the use of what they call 'time series methodologies', that is, recording changes in many different clients undergoing the same type of intervention over time, and once a substantial data set has been collected, looking for patterns, explanations and predictions of the changes that have occurred. A good example of this approach can be found in Beck's (1976) studies of cognitive therapy for clients with depression and anxiety problems. Establishing a comprehensive data set to compare different clients and their progress over time is essential. However, this does not resolve the problem of which intervention, background factors, client characteristics or type of client–therapist relationship determines an observable outcome.

There are two reasons why clinicians need to commit themselves to ongoing research and evaluation of their practice. The first is the obvious one: that not to engage in self-evaluation is to commit professional suicide. That is to say, to cease being interested and excited by growth and innovation is to lose an essential ingredient of good practice. The second reason is that 'professions that provide high quality services effectively and efficiently stay in business' (Minifie, 1983) whereas those that do not go bust. Frattelli (1990) made a similar point to her colleagues in the USA when she declared that 'If we do not collect these data (on our efficacy) policy makers outside the field will continue their current practice of arbitrarily making decisions without our input' (p.7). More recently, the UK Health Minister Virginia Bottomley, in an interview on Radio 4's 'World Tonight', said of the future of the National Health Service that 'the culture of caring and the culture of cost have got to be integrated'. If policy makers are to calculate accurately the cost of speech and language therapy services to people with learning disabilities, then speech and language therapy services must be able to describe what they are providing, for how long, and for what purpose.

There are already many instances where policy decisions about service delivery systems and clinical practices are based upon research outcomes. For example, in the UK the work of Lyle (1960), King et al. (1971) and others contributed to the change in government policy on institutional care for people with learning disabilities. Likewise, research on the importance of the pragmatic aspects of language (Bates, 1976) has influenced therapeutic practice. However, there is relatively little in the way of published research which examines the relative merits or demerits of different types of communication intervention with adults with learning disabilities. This is reflected in the number of published articles in the popular journals. For example, between 1978 and 1992, the British [now European] Journal of Disorders of Communication contained only seven articles that related specifically to research on the communication difficulties of adults with learning disabilities.

Research Methodologies

Having established that there is a need for more research into the communication skills of adults with learning disabilities, we turn to the question of how it can be achieved, and by whom. Seigel and Spradlin (1985), among others, have argued that research and clinical practice are very different pursuits, and require different skills. We would argue that this is not the case: there are strong parallels between research methods and therapeutic practices which can and indeed must be interwoven if the knowledge base on communication and learning disability is to increase. This may involve an element of demystifying research and evaluation, but is essential if health services professions are to survive in the current climate of accountability and 'value for money'.

In Chapter 8, we discussed some of the ways in which speech and language therapy services to adults with learning disabilities could be evaluated, for example by establishing specific entry and exit criteria for intervention, measuring change through the use of a variety of goal planning techniques and evaluating specific 'priorities for change' for each individual over a set time period. There are other methodologies: randomised controlled trials, quasi-experimental designs, single case studies and ethnographic designs, some of which can be successfully incorporated into clinical practice, whereas others are either difficult to implement or require commitments of time over and above that available to busy practitioners.

Randomised controlled trials

The ideal method for a controlled evaluation is the randomised controlled trial (Cochrane, 1972). This sets up an experimental situation (e.g. treatment method A) and a control situation (treatment method B, or no treatment at all) and randomly allocates clients to one of these two groups. As Abrahamson (1979) points out, 'randomisation does not guarantee that the experimental and control groups will be identical, but it reduces the influence of extraneous factors by ensuring that the only differences between the groups will be those which occur by chance'.

Practically, it is seldom possible to introduce a randomised controlled trial in everyday clinical practice. Clinicians tend to be reluctant to have their clients managed by chance and, quite rightly, invoke ethical considerations. These are mainly that clients allocated to the control group might be disadvantaged by not gaining the perceived or to-be-proven advantages of being in the experimental group. Alternatively, clinicians may fear that the unknown outcomes of the experimental treatment may be detrimental to their clients. Another

concern of clinicians is that randomisation takes away the consideration of clients' individual and particular needs, wants and expectations.
This is often seen as a breach of the professional–client relationship.

A randomised controlled trial also has practical problems. In particular, it is often very difficult, if not impossible, to organise the flow and
distribution of clients to the experimental and control groups on a randomised basis. This is particularly so in treatment settings which are
staffed by only one clinician (as is the case with many speech and language therapy services in the UK). The solution may involve those
clients randomised into the control group being treated by a different
therapist in a different locale, or on a different day. Both of these
options may be highly impractical for people who are physically or
intellectually disabled, who have transport difficulties or who cannot
be as flexible as a randomised controlled trial requires. It also under-
mines the notion of clients' choice and rights.

Even where randomised controlled trials have been undertaken in
health services research they may present problems of clinical relevance and ecological validity. For instance, the Northwick Park randomised controlled trial of physiotherapy (Smith et al., 1978) had to
exclude 89% of the hospital's stroke population ($n=1094$) on the
grounds that 20% died while in hospital, 30% were fully recovered
when discharged and 39% were too frail or ill to be considered for
inclusion in the trial. Although Smith et al. did find a dose–response
relationship between intensity of physiotherapy and outcome, this was
based on only 11% of the hospital population. This raises important
questions about the representativeness of those patients who were
included in the trial and, therefore, about the clinical relevance and
real-life validity of the study's findings.

In light of these and other problems associated with randomised
controlled trials (Illsley, 1980; Coulter, 1991) health service researchers
have utilised other methodologies. These have included quasi-experimental designs, single case studies and ethnography.

Quasi-experimental designs

Quasi-experimental designs are one solution to the problem of undertaking randomised controlled trials in that they encompass designs in
which random allocation of subjects is not a requirement (Cook and
Campbell, 1979). In all other respects, quasi-experimental designs con-
form to the same requirements as the controlled trial. Instead of random allocation, quasi-experimental designs use controlled before and
after measures, or compare two settings, using carefully matched
groups. In order to determine the long-term efficacy of an intervention,
and to ensure that observed changes are neither ephemeral nor the
consequence of the research process itself, A–B–A designs are some-

times used. Retrospective studies would also come under the category of quasi-experimental design, for example, where subjects in one group who received a new type of intervention are compared with a group who had received an older, more traditional type of intervention (Benson et al., 1985; Haywood and Switzky, 1985; Coolidge et al., 1986).

Quasi-experimental designs are more time-consuming and more difficult to conduct in the context of everyday clinical practice than single case studies. However, they are extremely valuable to practitioners, particularly in establishing the efficacy of intervention. The main weakness of quasi-experimental designs is that the results are almost always open to a number of possible interpretations. This is because the presence of variables other than the independent variable may have influenced the outcome. For example, in an A-B-A design, in which subjects are offered therapy A, followed by a period of no therapy (B), followed by more of therapy A, there is no way of being certain that the improvement was due to some factor other than the intervention itself. However, as Parry and Watts (1989) point out, a series of trials using therapy A can eventually determine which factors are most likely to have brought about change. Like the single case study, this type of design is much closer to real working practices than the RCT designs and therefore has much more social validity for practitioners.

Single case study designs

There can be little doubt that single case study designs have contributed greatly to the study of communication disorders. One of the most well known single case studies in the field of communication and learning disability was Curtiss' study of 'Genie', a 12-year-old girl who was discovered after living for years in a state of emotional and social deprivation (Curtiss, 1977). This detailed account of Genie's language development gave psycholinguists and practitioners new insights into language learning and social experience. Curtiss and her colleagues also undertook a series of studies on the communicative abilities of three young adults with learning disabilities (Curtiss et al., 1981). These studies reported interesting examples of apparent dissociations between the various subcomponents of language. For example, one young adult appeared to have more competence in the area of phonological and syntactic rules of language than in the area of lexical and semantic function. These and other single case studies of children with similar communicative patterns (for example, Blank et al.,1979; McTear, 1985) have contributed much to our knowledge and understanding of language.

Another widely known single case study of an adult's conversational abilities (Owings et al., 1981) suggested that conversational skills were to some extent dependent upon setting and familiarity with the conversational partner. Such studies have had considerable influence on practitioners' awareness of how important the characteristics of conversational settings can be.

More recently, O'Connor and Hermelin (1987), O'Connor (1989), and Hermelin and O'Connor (1990) have undertaken a series of case studies of 'idiot savants', individuals with learning disabilities who also have islets of outstanding ability. For example, these individuals may have outstanding memories for timetables, or map reading, or they may have exceptional musical or artistic abilities, despite having limited communication and social skills. These studies of the characteristics and capabilities of idiot savants have served as a challenge to what O'Connor (1989) called 'our complacent acceptance of generalised notions of intelligence and forced us to think again about the structure of the mind' (p.19).

Single case studies can be undertaken in the context of everyday clinical practice. Despite this, there have to date been few (published) single case studies of adults with learning disabilities generated by therapists in the UK compared, for example, with the number of studies generated by therapists working in areas such as aphasia or developmental language disorders.

Ethnographic designs

Ethnography differs from the methods described above in a number of ways. Goetz and LeCompte (1984) suggest that the purpose of ethnography is to provide descriptive data about the contexts, activities and beliefs of a group or groups of individuals. The roots of ethnography lie in anthropology, which has relied almost entirely upon the observational techniques now used in sociological, educational and psychological ethnography. The methods used differ markedly from those used in experimental research, in that ethnographers will collect naturalistic data and then use them to describe and analyse particular activities and interactions. Ethnographers generate categories of analysis, and give explanations as to the relationships between those categories. They use a combination of interviews and observations, using both audio and video recordings. Ethnographic enquiry may be based upon 'participant' or 'non-participant' observations. Participant observation is the involvement of researchers in the lives of those they are studying, often for long periods of time (Edgerton, 1967; Turner, 1982; Goode, 1983, 1984 and see below).

One of the difficulties of ethnographic designs is that data collection and analysis of this nature is very time-consuming. A great deal of data are generated by such detailed observations and this requires systematic and rigourous organisation and analysis. The methodological challenge

is for researchers to provide sufficiently detailed observations of particular activities in particular contexts, and to provide readers and other
analysts with the means of verifying or challenging the interpretation
and analysis that is being offered. This usually requires the researcher
to provide extensive field notes and other means of data collection,
often in the form of lengthy appendices.

An alternative means of undertaking detailed ethnography, and of
providing other researchers and readers with the means of verifying or
challenging what is being claimed or argued, is made possible by the
use of audio and, especially video, recordings of the activities under
investigation. Mehan (1979) has used the term 'constitutive ethnography' to characterise the systematic study of how everyday activities are
structured or constituted interactionally. Mehan's constitutive ethnography of classroom interactions involved video-taping the daily round
of classroom activities both obtrusively (i.e. with researchers operating
the video cameras in the classroom) and unobtrusively (i.e. by leaving
the video cameras recording unattended). The latter is one means of
avoiding another problem of participant observation and ethnography,
namely investigator bias (Edgerton, 1984b) or the Hawthorn effect; this
is the influence that the presence of researchers may have on the natural order of whatever is being investigated.

Mehan's video-taped recordings of classroom interactions were
played back to participants in the classroom (e.g. teachers), and to
other researchers, in order to elicit their responses and analyses of
what was going on. Mehan claims that this technique has the advantage
of providing representative materials of classroom activities over a period of time. It also allows the observational data to be retrieved for
exhaustive analysis by many researchers or analysts. A further advantage is that it facilitates a convergence between researchers' and participants' perspectives and allows an interactional level of analysis.

Mehan's approach has been used in other educational, medical
(Fisher, 1983; Todd, 1983) and psychiatric (Davies, 1979) settings. It
has also been used to study the professional competence of speech and
language therapists in the UK (see below) and as a more general means
of determining professional competence and quality assurance in the
caring professions (Caves, 1988).

Ethnography is based on the premise that behaviour is socially and
situationally constituted. In this respect it is unlike experimental
research, which assumes that there are universal principles of behaviour. In experimental research, these so-called universal principles are
investigated under controlled conditions, in which the influence of one
set of variables upon another is carefully measured. The outcome of
this measurement can then be generalised to the non-tested members
of the population only because the researchers accept that universal
principles of behaviour exist in the first place. Ethnographers make no

such assumptions in their study of behaviour. Anderson (1988) describes the techniques used by ethnographers as ways of uncovering meanings' the meanings which participants give to a situation, as well as the meanings that grow out of the situation as a whole' (p. 292). This process has been described as 'triangulation' : the collection of a variety of data, as well as the collection of multiple interpretations of the data. Glaser and Strauss (1967) compare it to the way in which surveyors will locate different points on a map.

Ethnography and people with learning disabilities

The study of people with learning disabilities has been greatly enhanced by ethnographic methods, particularly those of Robert Edgerton and his colleagues at the University of California, Los Angeles (Edgerton, 1963, 1967; Edgerton and Dingman, 1964; Zetlin and Sabsay, 1980; Turner, 1982; Goode, 1983, 1984; Graffam, 1983; Anderson Levitt and Platt, 1984; Sabsay and Platt, 1984;Sabsay and Platt, 1985). This work has been concerned with describing the lives of adults with mild to moderate learning disabilities living and working in a variety of settings. Much of it has been concerned with the communicative styles that individuals and groups use in the different settings. Conversation is viewed by all these researchers as a social as well as linguistic accomplishment and, as such, it is culturally defined (Brenneis, 1982). The researchers come from a wide variety of disciplines; sociology, anthropology, psycholinguistics, psychology and psychiatry. It is this variety of background experience that has given so much information, insight and understanding to the field of learning disabilities.

A particular contribution of this work is the way in which ethnographic studies can reveal what other research methods fail to do, or do much less successfully. In particular, ethnographic studies in the field of learning disabilities have identified abilities, competencies and dimensions of learning-disabled people which were not recognised by other methods of enquiry. A good example of this is Kernan and Turner's (1986) ethnographic study of the dream narratives of a group of adults with mild learning disabilities in a sheltered workshop setting. The study was part of a 3-year longitudinal study of life in the workshop. Kernan and Turner took part in weekly discussion groups in which participants had an opportunity to talk about their dreams. The researchers recorded and transcribed these weekly conversations, and examined their structure and content. They observed that the dream narratives were consistently being used to explore otherwise taboo subjects such as death and sex. The following is an account by one of the members of the group of one of his dreams:

'I was sleeping and my mother and father [both deceased] was in my room. A horrible dream. I heard her calling to me, 'Come, come.' I guess she wants me to go up there with her in heaven. I'm not ready yet.'

Kernan and Turner suggest that this kind of narrative allowed the individual to express the anxiety and grief that he was feeling. Outside the group, Kernan and Turner observed that similar attempts to talk about such 'bad' dreams are frequently rejected with comments from peers, 'just don't think about it', or 'behave like a grown up'. In the dream narrative group, however, the anxiety and grief is 'allowed', and the group often end up crying together when dreams like this one are related by individual members. Dreams in this context become a safe vehicle for talking about a taboo subject.

Kernan and Turner also observed that the group used dreams to sanction certain kinds of relationships, for example certain friendships between members of the group, and to entertain. Once the group became an established forum for discussing dreams, group-constructed dream narratives began to emerge, whereby members contributed to each others' dreams. During one session, a woman introduced a dream about a fancy dress party in which all group members had roles as various items of food, mostly fruit and vegetables. The dream was developed by the group, with different members adding stories about swimming parties, bikinis and various sexual escapades. The findings of this study contrasted with previous attempts to describe dream narratives (Walsch, 1920; De Martino, 1954; Sternlicht, 1966), which concluded that the dream reports of adults with learning disabilities were 'spare and impoverished, lacking in detail and richness or symbolism'. These earlier studies all used one-off interviews in which individuals were asked (by a stranger) to report any dreams they could recall. Not surprisingly, this method produced very few data and consequently arrived at very different conclusions.

Ethnographic studies have identified the setting in which communication takes place as central to the study of communication. Conversation involves weighing up social as well as linguistic factors in deciding what to say and how to say it. Turner (1982) suggests that the settings in which people find themselves engender their own set of 'communicative rules', which can only be identified through in-depth observation of the interactions that take place within those settings. Anderson Levitt and Platt (1984) and Platt (1985) used similar ethnographic techniques to describe the conversations of adults with similar degrees of mild learning difficulties in different settings. Anderson Levitt and Platt studied conversations that took place in a weekly peer counselling group at a sheltered workshop. Sabsay and Platt studied mealtime conversations in a group home for six women. The meal time conversations revolved around attempts by the women to display knowledge about a particular subject, even when the information had already been communicated by another member.

The following conversation took place on a Tuesday. It had rained the previous Tuesday, but was fair on this day.

Grace: Last week Tues - last Tuesday's raining not this Tuesday not
                raining.
Marcy: I know ((pause)) // It was nice.]
Elaine: // It sure was nice out today.]
Marcy: It was nice.
Carol: I know last Tuesday was raining', // I know.]
Elaine: //Who] else needs ice?

Platt pointed out that this type of communicative behaviour would be seen as a violation of one of Grice's (1975) basic conversational maxims: that speakers do not use their turn to provide information that listeners already know. In contrast, Anderson Levitt and Platt's study of conversation in a different setting found no examples of such a violation. Platt suggests that the reason for this discrepancy is contextually driven, that the rules of conversation vary from one context to another. In the group home, the major goals and preoccupations centred around establishing competence in household tasks and daily living skills. This desire to establish competence determined the pattern of the interactions that took place between the women. In contrast, the peer counselling group had completely different set of goals, and these too influenced the pattern of interactions that characterised the group.

Goode's ethnographic studies (1983, 1984) have provided new insights into the competencies of people with learning disabilities by undertaking what he calls an 'emic', rather than an 'etic' level of analysis. An 'etic' level of analysis is that which is provided from an outsider's perspective and which claims the status of being 'objective', detached and 'scientific'. It is the type of analysis that is often associated with a clinical perspective. An 'emic' level of analysis is that which is provided from an insider's perspective, or from the point of view of the person or people under investigation. This type of analysis focuses on the 'subjective', the experiential and the interpretive–hermeneutic levels of inquiry. In a series of studies, Goode has attempted to go beyond the etic level of analysis found in clinical reports, case notes and professional documents on people with learning disabilities. These, says Goode, tend to provide only deficit, or fault-finding, views of the people in question. By way of contrast, an 'emic' analysis not only provides a view of learning disabilities from the individuals' perspectives, but also identifies abilities and competencies which are often hidden from an 'etic' perspective.

An example of Goode's 'emic' analysis of people with learning difficulties is provided in his paper 'Who is Bobby?' (Goode, 1983). Bobby was a 50-year-old man with Down's syndrome who lived at a board and care facility (residential home with day care facilities) for people with learning disabilities. Goode notes that the view of Bobby gained from reading his case notes is essentially negative, fault-finding and deficit driven. Consider the following excerpts from Bobby's medical, speech and language therapy, clinical psychology and occupational therapy notes:

Medical assessment: diabetes with peripheral vascular disease.Oedema of the lower extremities.

Communication assessment: speech or language therapy is not recommended as prognosis for improvement is poor.... Client can communicate basic needs but cannot express complex ideas and understands very little.... Difficult to communicate with.

Cognitive assessment: a quick test of intelligence yielded a mental age of approximately 2;8 years. Clinician concludes that Bobby is 'severely mentally retarded with severe brain damage'.

Occupational therapy assessment: time and effort in this area are not suggested as prognosis for improvement is poor.... Maintain client in a protected environment as he can never function independently.

Goode points out that Bobby's communication *was* difficult to understand. The issue that arises is whether this is all that could be said about Bobby and whether, by doing so, clinicians were in fact failing to identify Bobby's abilities and competencies in different contexts. Goode found, for instance, that as a participant observer he was able to see Bobby within his peer group and in a variety of situations. In these contexts Goode found that Bobby was able to communicate very well with his peers, and they with him. Within the home Bobby was said to have 'no communication problems' and to have 'talked fine'. Indeed, it was pointed out to Goode by the other residents of the home that 'you (the researchers) just didn't understand him'.

Over time, Goode came to appreciate these views of Bobby and to acquire the communicative and cognitive ability to understand and to view him as someone who could express his thoughts and feelings. Goode observed, for instance, that Bobby produced semantically meaningful utterances using a limited range of syntactic structures, and that he recognised and responded to the illocutionary force of speech acts (e.g. requests, commands, greetings). Observations of Bobby in his own social environment indicated that he was understood by his communicative partners and that he understood much of what went on around him. Bobby's other abilities included being humorous and recognising humour, arguing and taking a position in a conversation, recognising other people's positions and strategies in an argument and being capable of abstract thought (such as recognising the meaning of privacy).

One reason why there were discrepancies between the clinical ('etic') and the peer-group ('emic') views of Bobby was that the former were generated in the formal and rather alien context of clinics, whereas the latter were formed in the more relaxed setting of Bobby's home and everyday environment. Goode's ethnographic notes and video tapes indicated that within the clinic Bobby was tense, lacked confidence, was frustrated at not being understood, did not participate and, when he did speak, enunciated poorly and failed to project his voice. By way of contrast, when Bobby was with his friends at home he was more relaxed, more assured, more knowledgeable about the affairs going on around him, more willing to volunteer remarks and pro- nounced utterances more clearly and forcefully. This reinforces the importance not only of assessing individuals' communicative environ- ment (see Chapter 4) but of doing this across the range of contexts in which they live and communicate. It also suggests that integrating ethnographic methods into clinical assessment and practice could bear much fruit.

Ethnographic studies of people with learning disabilities have also focused on the interactional and conversational strategies of carers. Sabsay and Platt (1984) for instance, demonstrated how carers develop compensatory strategies with certain individuals whom they judge to be 'incompetent' in certain conversational settings. For example, they may overcompensate for an individual by taking over when the individ- ual appears to be failing to relate the details accurately. Some carers have more insight than others that they are doing this. One carer described it thus:

> There are many times in conversation when I get used to the feeling Marilyn just plain doesn't understand. I'm so used to it I immediately compensate for it by rescuing it with a small explanation or rewording, saving her from ever having to admit she doesn't understand.

> (Sabsay and Platt, p.14)

This is consistent with Edgerton's (1967) observation that those who interacted with people who have learning difficulties also engaged in a 'benevolent conspiracy' to avoid embarrassing them, for instance, not revealing that they were aware of their communicative inabilities.

Another strategy commonly observed (Linder, 1978; Sabsay and Platt, 1984) is that carers may undercompensate, making the individual appear less competent than he or she actually is. Take this example from Linder (1978) from a conversation about G's recent stay at a sum- mer camp:

M: And how about dinner?
G: I had some spaghetti.
M: Did you like that?
G: Yes.
M: You like spaghetti?
G: Great!

This very short exchange suggests that this kind of response does not give the client any opportunity to expand or develop his narrative. Ethnographic data such as these often reveal an impoverished communication environment in which one must ask whether the full abilities and competencies of people with learning disabilities can be stimulated, nurtured and developed. This, once again, endorses the view that learning disabilities may be as much a feature of the environment and context in which people live and interact as it is about their supposedly innate cognitive and communicative abilities.

This type of research is rare among speech and language therapists in the UK, yet it has demonstrated that it can provide the kind of detail necessary to develop new ways of working with adults with learning disabilities. It provides the examples that are essential to understanding the patterns that exist. It provides new insights into the communication skills of adults with learning disabilities. Most of the work that has been done by the Socio Behavioural Group at UCLA has concentrated on adults with mild to moderate disabilities. The gap in terms of research is now in the area of the interactions of people who have more limited verbal communication skills.

Aylwin (1988) suggested that practitioners may, in theory, be sympathetic to the use of such qualitative research techniques, but they may not find appropriate descriptions of how it is actually carried out in practice. In view of this, a recent ethnographic study of speech and language therapists working with adults with learning disabilities is described in detail below.

Ethnographic study of everyday clinical practice in speech and language therapy

Rationale for the study

The purpose of this study was to examine speech and language therapists' perceptions of their own knowledge and skills base in the context of everyday clinical practice. It compared the knowledge and skills identified in a much larger consultative study of speech and language therapists' competence (van der Gaag and Davies, 1992a, b; Davies and van der Gaag, 1992a, b) with the knowledge and skills identified by four speech and language therapists working with adults with learning disabilities, reflecting on a 'typical' day in their working lives.

The consultative study examined the competence of speech and language therapists working with three client groups: the elderly, children and people with learning difficulties. In order to determine which knowledge, skills and attitudes were essential to the competence of the therapist, the authors consulted 67 speech and language therapy 'experts': clinicians and academics who were considered expert by their peers. The items of knowledge and skill generated by the experts were then distributed among 657 speech and language therapists specialising in work with one of the three client groups. These specialists were asked to confirm or reject whether each item on the list was essential, desirable or irrelevant to the competence of a speech therapist. The items on the lists were then rank ordered according to the level of agreement reached by the returns from the specialists. The majority of the items generated by the experts were confirmed as relevant to professional competence by the specialists (see Appendices I–XIII).

The consultative study concluded that speech and language therapy had a broad base, incorporating knowledge and skills from many different disciplines. However, questions remained about the relevance of these items to everyday clinical practice. Were all the knowledge and skills generated by the experts and agreed on by the specialists really being used on a day to day basis? Were there differences between what therapists reported was essential to professional competence, and what they actually did in practice? Van der Gaag and Davies (1992a) suggested that consultative methods alone could not identify those items of knowledge or skill which were present in everyday clinical contexts. They therefore decided to use ethnographic techniques in order to establish more precisely which knowledge and skill items were being used by therapists on a day to day basis.

Methods used in the study

Four speech and language therapists specialising in work with people with learning disabilities were asked to select a day in their working lives which they felt was 'typical', i.e. which included activities and routines that featured regularly in their work. They were then asked to select one or more ways of recording their everyday work activities.These were the diary method, the observational method and the video method.

Diary method

Therapists kept a detailed record of the day's activities, and would then identify for each activity what knowledge and skills they were using.

Observation method

One of the researchers spent a day with the therapist, recording the details of each activity and then asking the therapist to identify what knowledge and skills she was using for each.

Video method

This method, referred to as interpersonal process recall (Kagan, 1984);

involves recording the day's activities on video, and then asking the therapist to analyse each activity.

All four therapists opted for the observation method. In addition, two of them chose to use the video method for a small selection of activities which they felt to be representative of their work: one chose to analyse a video tape of a session which had been observed by one of the researchers; the other chose to analyse a pre-recorded video tape of her work.

Recall of knowledge and skills

Having recorded the therapists' work activities in the above ways, each therapist was asked to recall the work she had undertaken. Where necessary, the researcher gave her a resumé of the day's activities. She was then asked to specify, for each activity, what knowledge and skills she thought she had used. These items were recorded verbatim.

Recall with prompt

Following her recall of knowledge and skills, the therapist was then asked to review her day's work using the list of knowledge and skill items generated by the experts and specialist speech and language therapists (see Appendices I–XIII). She was asked to select the main activities of the day, for example, a group therapy session, an individual therapy session, a meeting with care staff, a lecture to nursing students, and identify the knowledge and skill items on the list which she felt she had used for each activity.

Recall with video

For this method, the therapist and researcher watched the video tape of the therapy session. As they did so, both were at liberty to stop the tape at any time and comment, or ask questions about the interactions (Davies, 1979; Mehan, 1979). Specifically, the researcher would ask the therapist to explain what knowledge and skills she was using at particular junctures in the therapy session.

These methods could be employed in other contexts, such as the evaluation of staff training, or the evaluation of specific intervention techniques used individually or with groups of clients. Some of these techniques have been used as intervention strategies as well. For example, interpersonal process recall has been used extensively in training students in the use of interpersonal skills. For more detailed accounts of the use of this technique, the reader is referred to Kagan (1984).

Results of the study

Sixty-five per cent of knowledge items and 76% of the skill items listed

Table 9.1 Comparison between knowledge and skill domains generated by consultative vs ethnographic studies of speech and language therapists' competence

Knowledge domains	Total number of items in consultative study	Total number of items included in both studies	% of items included in both studies (rounded to nearest whole figure)
Speech and Language	11	11	100
Psychology	13	8	61
Medical	12	9	75
Educational*	7	2	28
Policy	7	4	57
Assessment	9	7	78
Management	7	6	86
Knowledge specific to working with adults	16	6	38
Total	82	53	X % = 65%
Skill domains			
Therapeutic/teaching	32	26	81
Psychological	8	7	87
Speech/language	7	5	71
Management	19	12	63
Total	66	50	X % = 76%

* Only one speech and language therapist was working in the school setting in the ethnographic study

by the experts were named by one or more of the four therapists in the study. Many of the items generated by the panel of experts in the consultative study were also named, quite spontaneously, by the speech and language therapists as they reflected on the knowledge and skills they felt they were using in an everyday clinical context. Table 9.1 presents a comparison of the knowledge and skill items generated by consultative methods with those items generated using ethnographic techniques.

The strongest level of agreement between items generated by the experts and those named by the four therapists was in the speech and language domain (100% agreement). The lowest level of agreement on skills was in the educational domain. There was, however, only one therapist in the ethnographic study who worked exclusively in school settings.

There were additional items generated by the four therapists, all of them linked in some way to the items generated by the panel of experts. Some of these were specific examples of therapeutic or teaching skills. For example, one therapist mentioned knowledge of modelling techniques, role reversal and Knill techniques (examples of specific therapeutic techniques). All these were very specific to the day's activities. Another therapist had been to visit a residential home for people with learning difficulties for the first time, and she felt that she had used her skills in 'selling the speech and language therapy service to the staff in the home'. This kind of 'public relations' work was not mentioned by the panel of experts, although the experts may have argued that it was subsumed under some other heading, such as staff training training carers (see Appendix I).

It was interesting to note that 30 items were generated by the experts which were not mentioned by any of the therapists. These included knowledge of autism, emotional disturbance, psychotherapeutic approaches, and drug use/misuse (Table 9.2)

In order to discover more about the discrepancies between the experts and the therapists, the researchers consulted each of the therapists about the knowledge and skill items that they had not mentioned at the recall stage. They were asked to comment on each item. There appeared to be a strong consensus as to why these items had not been mentioned: the therapists said that some of these items were not relevant to the clients seen on the day. For example, knowledge of autism was not mentioned because none of the therapists saw clients who were autistic. When they were asked if they thought that such knowledge was essential to working with people with learning difficulties, they all agreed that it was. The same applied to emotional disturbance, psychotherapeutic approaches, drug use and misuse. For example, none of the clients seen were on any medication, but others in the caseload were receiving medication of some sort. Similarly, with test interpretation, no tests were being used at the time. The same interpretation was applied to the items listed by the experts relevant to elderly people with learning difficulties. None of the therapists saw elderly clients on those days.

A few of the items were not identified because therapists were unsure of the terminology used by the experts. A few more were not mentioned because they were not considered relevant to everyday clinical practice. These were psychological assessments, the role of voluntary agencies, local and national policies. The remaining items not identified by the therapists fell into one of two categories: either they were not considered necessary below management level, for example, quality assurance issues, or they were items which therapists said they simply 'took for granted' as part of their knowledge and skills base. For example, awareness of parents' rights, the school routine, classroom practices, and issues surrounding sexuality and handicap were all included in this.

Table 9.2 Breakdown of items listed by experts in the consultative study but *not* appearing in knowledge and skills analysis by speech and language therapists in the ethnographic study

---

Knowledge items

Psychology:	Autism (1)
	Emotional disturbance (1)
	Holistic approaches (3)
	Psychotherapeutic approaches (1)
	Psychological assessments (4)
Medical:	Drug use/abuse/misuse (1)
	Epidemiology of mental handicap (2)
	Diagnostic processes e.g. genetic testing(4)
Educational:	Statementing (2)
	Educational resources available (6)
	Parent's rights (6)
	The school routine (6)
	Classroom practices (6)
Policy:	Community mental handicap teams (6)
	The role of voluntary agencies (4)
	Local and national policies (4) (6)
Assessment:	Test interpretation (1)
	Specific language problems (1)
Management:	Discharge criteria (1)

Additional knowledge relevant specifically to adults
Acquired disorders of communication (1)
Communication strategies used in the elderly population (2)
Psychosocial/emotional development in adolescence/adulthood (6)
The psychology of ageing (2)
Sexuality and handicap (6)
Characteristics of CVA, degenerative conditions etc. (1)
Causes and symptoms of mental illness (1)
The ageing process (2)
Adult education (1)
Employment opportunities, training schemes (1)

Interpretation
1. Not relevant to clients seen on the day
2. Not relevant to age groups
3. Not widely used terminology
4. Not considered central to everyday clinical practice
5. Not necessary below management grade
6. Not part of 'logic in use' (knowledge taken for granted)

The number after each item indicates the explanation given by the therapist as to why the item was not included. CVA = cerebrovascular accident.

Recall with video

When therapists were asked to recall the knowledge and skills they were using in particular therapy sessions, they gave more detailed accounts of the therapeutic skills they were using, and rather less about their knowledge base. For example, one therapist described how she was using a number of skills in conjunction with one another: skills in making ongoing judgements throughout the session about when to present the client with new material, how much time to give the client to look at objects placed in front of him, monitoring the client's level of attention, guiding the client's attention back to the task when necessary, using reinforcers (both negative and positive) appropriately, deciding when to use signs, and looking at the difference the use of signs made to the client's comprehension of the task. This kind of detail was not generated through the earlier large-scale consultative methodologies.

This study used ethnographic techniques to describe the knowledge and skills of speech and language therapists working with people with learning disabilities. In doing so, it tried to understand more fully the nature of competence in everyday clinical practice. The kind of detail provided by studies such as this one demonstrates the value and versatility of ethnographic techniques. This is not to say that other research methodologies which utilise an entirely different approach are any less valuable in the search for new insights into communication and learning disabilities. No one method can claim superiority over any other. Aylwin (1988) and Levy (1988) both emphasise this in their discussions of the use of qualitative research methods. What is important is that a variety of methods are applied so that the richness and diversity in the lives and experiences of adults with learning disabilities can be explored more fully. There is much work to be done.

Chapter 10
Conclusions

The main aim of this book has been to explore connections between ideas and concepts from several disciplines and to put them into the context of communication and learning disabilities. This has, we hope, served as an introduction to those not yet familiar with current theories, and as a point of reference for those who are experienced in the field.

The book has a number of distinct sections but there is one theme which runs throughout its pages. This is that any assessment or intervention process used to enhance or to understand communication skills in adults with learning disabilities must be multidimensional in its approach. It must involve carers and other professionals, taking into account their views and motivations. It must look at communication skills in context and approach intervention in an eclectic way.

There remains a great deal to be done in terms of our understanding of the nature of communication and how we can assess it. There is also much more to be learnt about the lives and experiences of people with learning disabilities and how these experiences can influence communication. A third area of concern is how we as professionals can be most effective in enhancing the quality of life of individuals with communication difficulties.

The early part of the book explored in some detail the problems of communication assessment. For example, it re-examined the distinction between communication, language and linguistic communication. In the past, these terms have had a tendency either to be used synonymously or seen as completely separate. The result has been a lack of clarity in the purpose and process of assessment (see Chapter 2). This section also looked in detail at what makes communication effective. It argued that successful communication has much to do with the context and the participants as it is to do with the actual meaning of the gestures, words, signs or phrases that are being used. This by now well accepted theory (Bates, 1976; Owings and Guyette, 1982; Bedrosian,

1988; Morse, 1988), has important consequences for the process of communication assessment. One of the positive consequences of this multidimensional perspective on assessment has been that speech and language therapists and their colleagues have begun to look at communication in a more integrated way. It is now no longer generally accepted practice to assess only one aspect of an individual's communication in isolation. Instead, the assessor uses a multidimensional approach to assessment which involves looking at the individual's everyday communication experiences.

One of the negative consequences, however, is that the shift in focus has led many therapists to abandon assessment of the linguistic components of communication altogether. We have argued here that this is the outcome of therapists equating 'functional' with 'pragmatics', coupled with the lack of relevant and accessible linguistic models upon which to base any functional communication assessment strategy. In the third part of the book, Chapter 8 provides just such a strategy for examining communication in a functional way by correlating its formal and functional aspects. The strategy is not presented here as a substitute for existing communication assessments, many of which have excellent uses (see Chapter 4), but as a complementary model which is designed to enhance the multidimensional approach. The model is presented here for the first time, ready for practical application in the field, offered to practitioners as a more complete approach to assessment. It also points the way to further research into the psycholinguistic processes underlying the comunication skills of adults with learning disabilities.

The second part of the book continues with the same multidimensional theme. For example, Chapter 5 looks at the intervention process from three viewpoints: the client, the therapist and the communication environment. In order for intervention to be effective, we have argued that an in-depth perspective on the client's past experiences and how these may have influenced his or her communication skills is necessary. Adults with learning disabilities who have long-standing communication difficulties have frequently experienced negative feedback about their communication skills. They may have experienced rejection, social isolation or even victimisation by others. Another consideration is the therapist's perception of his or her role and persona in the intervention process. Of equal importance is the influence of the client's present experience of communication. The communication environment must therefore be given consideration when planning intervention. In the past, when communication assessment and intervention were more unidimensional, there was little thought given to the interactions between client and environment, client and therapist, and therapist and environment as they are described in this chapter. Good practice today, however, demands an interactive approach, which reflects a more realistic picture of what happens in everyday life. In Medawar's (1982) terms, it has become more a process of story telling than list writing.

In times of ever more limited resources, the intervention process itself cannot be separated from the wider issues of service delivery. This includes considering how best to deliver an effective service to as many individuals as possible. The book therefore examines service delivery in some depth. We suggest that, in order to work effectively in any context, the therapist must have an understanding of the culture in which she or he works. For this reason, we have looked at the history and philosophy of learning disabilities, including a section on normalisation and the advocacy movement. There are also examples of a range of day and residential services for those practitioners who have had little first-hand experience in this field. It is often the case that newly qualified therapists have had little exposure to these sorts of working environments.

Chapter 7 looked more specifically at speech and language service delivery issues. It asked: How can therapists use their limited time to greatest effect? How can they obtain maximum collaboration with carers and other professionals? How do they make decisions about which individuals require their services most urgently? How do they measure changes in their clients' communication skills? How do they measure their effectiveness in training carers? These are examples of the questions which surround effective service delivery. They are as much a part of intervention as the therapy itself.

The multidimensional theme continued through the illustrations of different working practices. These were intended to demonstrate the spectrum of intervention which exists within the field. Medawar (1982) suggested that imaginative and creative forces are at the heart of what scientists do. We asked in Chapter 1 whether speech and language therapists saw themselves and their work in this light. The examples of intervention described in these pages are surely evidence of that creativity and imagination. This variation in therapy is likely to expand still further as more therapists work in collaboration with carers and other professionals such as art, music, movement and drama therapists. There is little room in this scenario for a prescriptive approach advocating one therapeutic method for one 'type' of communication breakdown. Rather, the selection of an approach is influenced by external circumstances, such as the availability of other professionals, the knowledge and attitudes of the carers, and the needs, preferences and motivations of the client.

The final chapter of the book addressed some of the research issues most pertinent to communication and learning disabilities. We suggested that research questions are often overlooked by practitioners because they are perceived as 'someone else's problem', or issues 'to be left to researchers' We argued that there is an almost inevitable link between becoming more accountable and becoming more concerned with evaluative research. With the increasing demand for information on the effectiveness of services, there is an urgent need for more practitioner-based research.

The remainder of the chapter gave examples of different research methods. Its focus was on the use of ethnographic techniques which have been used successfully in the USA for many years. These studies have greatly enhanced our understanding of the everyday lives and communicative experiences of people with learning disabilities. Many practitioners will be aware of the great benefits of studying communication in depth, as part of a piece of work which can then be shared with other practitioners. Ethnography is one method of achieving this.

There is much work to be done. Until there is a more systematic documentation of which assessments and interventions are successful, and more analysis of why they are successful, there will continue to be a shortfall between the enthusiasm and commitment that therapists bring to their work in this specialty and finding the most effective ways of applying their expertise.

Useful Addresses

Advocacy

Values into Action (formerly Campaign for People with Mental
Handicaps) and People First
Oxford House
Derbyshire Street
London E2 6HG

Agencies

Association for Spina Bifida and Hydrocephalus
56 Camberwell Road
London E2 6HG

British Institute of Mental Handicap Resource Centre
Wolverhampton Road
Kidderminster
Worcs DY10 3PP

British Dyslexia Association
98 London Road
Reading

British Deaf Association
38 Victoria Place
Carlisle
Cumbria

British Sports Association for the Disabled
34 Osnaburgh Street
London NW1 3ND

Carers' National Association
29 Chilworth Mews
London W2 3RG

National Association for the Protection from Sexual Abuse of Adults and
Children with Learning Disabilities (NAPSAC)
Pam Cooke
Development Officer
Department of Mental Handicap
University of Nottingham Medical School
Queens Medical Centre
Nottingham NG7 2UH

National Autistic Society
276 Willesden Lane
London NW2 5BR

MENCAP National Centre
123 Golden Lane
London EC1Y 0RT

MIND (National Association for Mental Health) 22 Harley Street
London W1

Open University Education for Disabled Students
Po Box 79
Milton Keynes
MK7 6AA

Royal National Institute for the Blind
224 Great Portland Street
London W1A 4XX

Royal National Institute for Deaf People (RNID)
105 Gower Street
London WC1

The Spastics Society
12 Park Crescent
London W1N 4EQ

Assessments

NFER-Nelson
2 Oxford Road East
Windsor
Berkshire SL4 1DF

Forum Consultancy
Lucy Hurst Brown
St Mark's ATC
Ladbroke Grove
London W8

Speech Profiles
11b Winton Drive
Glasgow G12 OPZ

Complementary Therapies

The Association of Dance and Movement Therapy
99 South Hill Park
London NW4 2SP

British Association for Dramatherapists
PO Box 98
Kirbymoorside
Yorks YO6 6EX

British Society for Music Therapy
69 Avondale Ave
East Barnet
Herts
EN4 8NB

Jigsaw Dance Company
Cheryl Strong
Robert Owen Centre
4a Dale Avenue
The Murray, East Kilbride
Glasgow G 43

Aromatherapy Associates
68 Maltings Place
London SW6 2BY

International Federation of Reflexologists
78 Edridge Road
Croydon

British College of Acupuncture
8 Hunter Street
London WC1N 1BN

Social Skills Pack

Carole Charters and Lynn Drumm
Community Team for People with Learning Disabilities
Woodland Centre
Memorial Hospital
Hollyhurst Road
Darlington
Co. Durham DL3 6HX

Staff Training

Sue Whitefoot
Gorsty Cottage
St Michaels
Tenbury Wells
Worcestershire
WR15 8TW

Appendix I

Learning Disabilities

Distribution of agreement on the skills base of speech and language therapy for therapists working with children and adults with learning disabilities

Therapeutic teaching skills

	1	2	3	4
			(%)	
Selecting and using effective and appropriate techniques – including the following:				
Making a differential diagnosis (speech and language)	98	1	–	–
Knowing when to terminate therapy	93	5	1	–
Appropriate assessments	86	11	2	–
Interpreting data	85	12	2	–
Demonstration of therapeutic techniques	81	10	4	1
Program planning	72	19	8	–
In-depth observation skills	39	45	13	3
Changing the communication environment	27	30	27	12
Structuring a learning situation	19	61	14	5
Flexibility of presentation	19	44	23	12
Presentation of appropriate materials	10	15	47	24
Using/creating appropriate materials	5	20	47	24
Handling and positioning children appropriately	1	29	43	24
Using movement and drama techniques	–	32	36	27
Using artistic abilities	–	12	25	59
Clinical training of speech therapy students	92	6	1	–

*Percentages do not always add up to 100 because of missing values.

	1	2	3	4
		(%)		
Developing a shared perspective/establishing				
common goals – including the following:				
Ability to prioritise caseload with other				
professionals	68	24	3	1
Communicating therapy goals to carers	58	19	10	9
Matching expressive mode to that of client	29	10	32	24
Facilitating skills of carers	24	40	22	9
Facilitating communication in people with little				
or no communicative intent	22	15	37	20
Establishing rapport	6	10	17	61
Forming reciprocal relationships	5	10	20	59
Using reinforcers appropriately	5	17	44	–
Decision-making about interactive therapeutic				
procedures/establishing a therapeutic				
dialogue – including the following:				
Deciding on the correct timing of intervention	77	15	5	2
Deciding on the correct timing of presentation	48	30	14	6
Using vocabulary appropriately	24	12	32	27
Respond appropriately to a wide range of verbal				
and non-verbal communication	20	11	34	31
Cueing	19	19	39	23
Shaping	16	23	38	20
Carrying out sequenced programmes	7	4	41	43
Analysing/managing challenging behaviour	6	71	17	4

Appendix II

Learning Disabilities

Distribution of agreement on the skills base of speech and language therapy for therapists working with children and adults with learning disabilities.

Psychological skills

	1	2	3	4
		(%)		
Evaluating outcomes	55	37	3	2
Research skills, e.g. evaluate research literature	50	46	1	1
Counselling	24	67	4	2
Interpersonal skills – including the following:				
Explaining skills	32	42	13	11
Assessing others expectations	19	55	13	10
Listening skills	16	28	25	29
Observation skills	11	34	25	27
Motivating others	10	44	19	24

Appendix III

Learning Disabilities

Distribution of agreement on the skills base of speech and language therapy for therapists working with children and adults with learning disabilities.

Speech/language related skills

	1	2	3	4
		(%)		
Analysis of all aspects of communicative behaviour				
– including the following:				
Phonetic/phonemic transcriptions	97	1	1	–
Syntactic, semantic, pragmatic analyses	95	3	1	–
Pre-verbal communication behaviours	65	26	7	1
Use of augmentative/alternative systems,				
e.g. signed communication	53	19	13	14
Application of knowledge of computers	8	47	20	23
Application of knowledge of video recording	5	38	23	31
Chewing and swallowing abilities	77	19	3	–

Appendix IV

Learning Disabilities

Distribution of agreement on the skills base of speech and language therapy for therapists working with children and adults with learning disabilities.

Business and client management skills

	1	2	3	4
		(%)		
Working with speech and language therapy volunteers	65	18	8	7
Report writing	61	27	8	3
Readiness to work as an independent practitioner	61	25	3	3
Working with speech and language assistants	60	26	5	7
Goal planning	52	33	11	3
Coping with non-compliance from staff	49	42	4	3
Involvement in special interest groups	39	19	17	25
Active participation in policy-making	38	42	12	7
Involvement in IPPs	35	32	16	11
Supporting staff	32	40	15	13
Time-management skills	25	30	18	25
Running groups	25	20	42	11
Organisational skills	24	31	18	24
Problem-solving	20	38	24	14
Record-keeping	13	12	32	40
Appointment making	10	4	27	57
Helping clients to make choices	7	26	27	39
Helping carers to 'let go'	5	50	23	18
Maintaining and handling equipment	3	1	18	77

Appendix V

Learning Disabilities

Distribution of agreement on the skills base of speech and language therapy for therapists working with children and adults with learning disabilities.

Speech and language

	Essential	Desirable (%)	Irrelevant
Pre-linguistic development	98	1	–
Linguistic development	97	1	–
Speech and language delay/disorders	96	3	–
Syntax	92	7	–
Semantics	92	7	–
Phonetics/Phonology	89	9	–
Linguistic analyses – including:	80	14	–
Pragmatics	89	10	–
Semantics	85	14	–
Phonetics/Phonology	84	15	–
Syntax	84	14	–

Appendix VI

Learning Disabilities

Distribution of agreement on the knowledge base of speech and language therapy for therapists working with children and adults with learning disabilities.

Psychology

	Essential	Desirable (%)	Irrelevant
Normal child development	97	2	–
Cognitive development	94	5	–
Learning theories	78	21	1
Autism	75	24	–
Behaviour modification techniques	67	32	1
Emotional disturbance	65	33	–
Counselling techniques	62	37	–
Bereavement response to handicap	47	51	2
Holistic approaches	45	53	2
Psychological assessments	30	68	1
The acquisition of literacy skills	21	70	7
Psychotherapeutic approaches	17	76	6
The acquisition of numeracy skills	11	69	18

Appendix VII

Learning Disabilities

Distribution of agreement on the knowledge base of speech and language therapy for therapists working with children and adults with learning disabilities

Medical

	Essential	Desirable (%)	Irrelevant
Sensory impairment	95	4	–
Physical handicaps	87	12	–
Neurology	85	14	–
Hearing problems/audiological testing	83	17	–
Anatomy and physiology	75	22	–
Aetiology of mental handicaps	73	24	2
Medical conditions associated with mental handicaps	67	32	–
Specific syndromes and their characteristics	54	46	–
Management of epilepsy	48	48	2
Drug use/reactions/misuse	24	69	6
Epidemiology of mental handicap	21	66	11
Diagnostic processes, e.g. genetic testing	8	67	24

Appendix VIII

Learning Disabilities

Distribution of agreement on the knowledge base of speech and language therapy for therapists working with children and adults with learning disabilities.

Educational

	Essential	Desirable (%)	Irrelevant
Statementing	93	6	–
Educational resources available	76	23	1
Parents rights	75	24	–
The school routine	63	34	2
The National Curriculum	57	39	2
Classroom practice	56	42	1
Treatment techniques, e.g. Bobath, Peto	29	70	–

Appendix IX

Learning Disabilities

Distribution of agreement on the knowledge base of speech and language therapy for therapists working with children and adults with learning disabilities.

Policy

	Essential	Desirable (%)	Irrelevant
Community mental handicap teams	76	23	–
Principals of normalisation	71	26	2
Local and national policies, e.g. Warnock, Griffiths, Education Acts	62	37	1
Social attitudes to disability	56	41	1
Joint health, education and social services planning (e.g. funding issues, service delivery issues)	45	48	3
Social policies	39	56	3
Role of voluntary agencies	39	57	2

Appendix X

Learning Disabilities

Distribution of agreement on the knowledge base of speech and language therapy for therapists working with children and adults with learning disabilities.

Assessment

	Essential	Desirable (%)	Irrelevant
Specific speech and language assessments (including assessment of functional communication)	97	1	–
Test interpretation	96	3	–
Alternative/augmentative systems	95	3	–
Checklist assessments, (including feeding assessments)	94	54	–
Specific language problems	91	7	–
Assessment of the client's likes and dislikes	85	13	–
Techniques of linguistic analysis (including discourse analysis)	72	27	–

Appendix XI

Learning Disabilities

Distribution of agreement on the knowledge base of speech and language therapy for therapists working with children and adults with learning disabilities

Client management

	Essential	Desirable (%)	Irrelevant
Teaching functional communication skills	96	3	–
Alternative/augmentative techniques	96	3	–
Specific language programmes	90	9	1
Discharge criteria	89	9	1
Personal awareness/professional development (e.g. personal strengths and weaknesses, insight into in-service training needs etc.)	89	10	–
Multidisciplinary team approach	89	10	–
Management of chewing and swallowing problems	83	16	–

Appendix XII

Learning Disabilities

Distribution of agreement on the knowledge base of speech and language therapy for therapists working with children and adults with learning disabilities.

Additional knowledge relevant specifically to adults

	Essential	Desirable (%)	Irrelevant
Speech and Language			
Long term effects of speech and language problems	81	14	–
Acquired disorders of communication	71	23	2
Communication strategies in the elderly population	52	40	4
Psychology			
Lifestyles and their effects, e.g. effects of institutionalisation or community care	76	20	–
Psycho-social and emotional development in adolescence and adulthood	52	43	1
Handling violence	51	43	2
The psychology of ageing	40	54	2
Sexuality and handicap	30	56	10
Medical			
Characteristics of CVA, progressive neurological diseases, tumour, head injury and the dementias	65	29	1
Causes and symptoms of mental illnesses	47	46	3
Expectations of adulthood (e.g. good health, lifestyle)	39	48	6
The ageing process	39	54	2
Education and work			
Social services provision	47	47	2
Opportunities for further education	35	58	3
Adult education – policies	33	58	6
Employment opportunities, training schemes	33	57	5

Appendix XIII

Learning Disabilities

Distribution of agreement on the attitude base of speech and language therapy for therapists working with children and adults with learning disabilities.

	Essential	Desirable (%)	Irrelevant
Adaptable	96	3	–
A belief that communication is a basic right	94	4	1
Professionalism	93	5	–
Realistic	91	8	–
Ability to see the whole	91	8	–
A willingness to acquire new skills	90	9	–
Reliability	90	8	–
Positive	89	10	–
Interest in the work	89	10	–
A listening attitude	87	11	0.5
Ability to be a facilitator	86	13	–
Motivation	86	12	–
Empathy	80	20	–
Constructive	80	19	–
Enthusiasm	78	21	–
Discreet	77	19	3.0
Acceptance of own limitations	73	25	1.0
Persevering	73	23	2.0
Self awareness	70	30	–
Patience	70	25	3.0
To see the therapist as an agent of change	65	28	4.0
Sense of humour	62	36	1.0
A belief in the profession	61	33	4.0
Ability to compromise	56	40	2.0
Assertive	49	48	1.0
Non-defensive	49	46	3.0
Self confident	47	51	–
Tenacious	37	48	13
Thick skinned	22	35	39
Idealism	16	37	44

Appendix XIV

Therapists' Perceptions of their Own Knowledge and Skills Base Applied to Specific Clinical Practice

Therapist: A
Therapy: One-to-one with adult(s) with severe learning disabilities
Date: Feb. 91
Analysis: Recall with video

Knowledge

Domain	Client 1	Client 2
Speech and Language	Normal and abnormal communicative interactions – what is involved Linguistics – client's linguistic ability Preverbal communication Non-verbal communication – *body language, eye pointing	Preverbal communication Non-verbal communication Use of body language Linguistic ability of client Interaction
Psychology	Psychological theories Behaviourist principles *Levels of attention, concentration *Theories about the use of reinforcers	Knowledge of how to use demonstration and modelling techniques
Medical	Characteristics of Down's syndrome – speech production – signing/gestural manner – hearing problems	
Policy	Principles of normalisation Accepting clients for who they are	Normalisation principles

Domain	Client 1	Client 2
Assessment	Assessment procedures – which are appropriate, appropriate materials When to use signs, how to look at the difference they make to comprehension Signing theories, why signs are used Client's home background, linguistic experience *Assessment of imitation skills *How to decide on the need for more in-depth assessment, and in which areas	Signing theory, use of signs
Management	(As this was an assessment session, most items listed above) Signing techniques	Knowledge of specific therapeutic techniques * e.g. Knill techniques *Knowledge of the differences between directive and non-directive therapy *How to manage client with very severe comm. handicap How to manage client with CB *Knowledge of client/therapist relationship

Skills

Domain	Client 1	Client 2
Therapeutic/ teaching	Timing of presentation *giving the client time to look at objects in front of him *Monitoring attention level, bringing client's attention back to the task Making judgements throughout the session about language level, signing abilities Use of reinforcers (not being negative without being positive), Knowing when to be silent, when to speak, when to use signs	Structuring the therapy Giving appropriate non-verbal and verbal input Timing of presentation *Use of demonstration techniques *Use of modelling techniques How to follow client's comm. behaviour Using specific techniques movement, music techniques *Communicating with a client who has a very severe comm. handicap *How to get client's attention *How to be non-directive with client
Psychological	Indepth observation of all aspects of client's behaviour	
Speech/language	Use of signing techniques	Use of signing techniques
Management		Knowledge of client/ therapist relationship Managing challenging behaviour

Therapist: B
Therapy: Informal Staff Training
Date: Jan. 91
Analysis: Recall without prompt

Knowledge

Domain:	
Speech and language	Client's linguistic abilities in depth
Psychology	Counselling techniques Knowledge of client's abilities Bereavement response to handicap
Medical	Knowledge of client's medical history aetiology etc.
Educational	Teaching techniques – formal and informal methods
Policy	Aims and objectives of the speech therapy department, how to meet client needs in this context Principles of normalisation, advocacy
Assessment	Assessment procedures relevant to adults Knowledge of the client's environment Observation techniques
Management	Local facilities Using the multidisciplinary approach, liaising with others How to approach,deal with, staff

Skills

Domain:	

Therapeutic/teaching	Making judgements about the correct timing of
	  interactions with staff
	Making judgements about staff's level of interest,
	  motivation, level of knowledge

Psychological	Observation skills Listening skills Communication skills/interpersonal skills Negotiation skills Research skills
Speech and language	Assessment of clients: which ones need speech therapy Using formal and informal assessment procedures
Management	*How to 'sell' the speech therapy services Liaising with staff Negotiating with staff *Coping with stress

Therapist: C
Therapy: One to one with adult with learning disability
Date: Dec. 90
Analysis: Recall without prompt

Knowledge

Domain:	
Speech and language	Client's linguistic abilities, language functions
	Appropriate levels of linguistic ability
	Non-verbal communication
Psychology	Management of challenging behaviour
	Behaviour modification techniques
	Numeracy and literacy skills
	*Social skills
Medical	Medical background of the client
Policy	Principles of normalisation
Assessment	Assessment procedures
	Knowledge of the carer's expectations
	Assessment of the clients' abilities
Management	Setting objectives
	Programme planning
	Organisation of resources
	Management of speech therapy students
	Knowledge of computers
	Knowledge of sign and symbol systems, electronic aids
	Therapeutic techniques
	Task analysis
	Administrative tasks, e.g. filing, data recording
	Writing reports

Skills

Domain:	
Therapeutic/teaching	Managing challenging behaviour
	Teaching social/interactional skills
	Using reinforcers
	Using the community setting to achieve objectives
	Maintaining client's interest and motivation
	Managing the client in different settings
	Applying knowledge of the client's abilities
	Using computer software appropriately
Psychological	In depth observation skills
	Evaluation skills
	Problem solving skills
	Research skills
	Interactional skills (*including public speaking, telephone skills)
	*Skills in fund raising for equipment
Speech and language	Applying knowledge of sign and symbol systems appropriately
Management	Working with other professionals
	Working with other speech therapists

Preparing therapy materials
Planning and organising therapy
Administrative skills e.g. data collection
Maintenance of equipment, e.g. computers, communication aids
Teaching others, passing on information

Therapist: D
Therapy: Language group in school for children with severe learning disabilities
Date: Jan. 91
Analysis: Recall without prompt and recall with video

Knowledge

Domain:	Recall without prompt	Recall with video
Speech and language	Speech and language delays Speech and language – phonology, syntax, semantics, pragmatics development Non-verbal communication	Language development Language abilities of each child Communication skills
Psychology management	Normal child development Cognitive development (*including auditory development, and concep.development)	Behaviour management Emotional development and its effects on the child's language *Group dynamics *Auditory memory Cognitive development Problem solving
Medical	Management of epilepsy Medical background to each child Aetiology, medical history	The childrens' physical development Physical handicaps Hearing problems Visual problems
Educational	Teaching techniques	The National Curriculum Fitting into the school routine
Assessment	Speech and language abilities and general abilities – what to expect Specific language assessments e.g. DLS Signing: rationale for its use, how to use it	Use of Makaton Knowledge of Derbyshire Language scheme
Management	Administration tasks e.g. writing reports Planning intervention Training teachers to use signs Setting aims and	Specific therapeutic techniques, e.g. DLS Makaton techniques Knowledge of teachers and how to work with them

objectives   *Knowledge of role-reversal
Use of specific   techniques
   therapeutic techniques
    *e.g. role reversal
Use of video equipment
*Sorting through case notes

Skills

Domain:	Recall without prompt	Recall with video

Therapeutic/teaching	Setting appropriate tasks
	Using appropriate
	  language
	*Giving physical prompts
	Cueing
	Maintaining children's
	  attention
	Varying order of
	  presentation,
	  timing of presentation
	*Using role reversal
	Using reinforcers
	Using appropriate signs
	Providing children with
	  opportunities to
	  communicate
	*Prompting
	Facilitating specific
	  comm. functions
		Use of reinforcers
		Appropriate use of language/
		  signs for each child
		Managing children in groups
		*Use of role reversal
		*Keeping the group moving
		*Keeping children's interest
		Timing the activities
		  appropriately
		*Making judgements about
		  when to bring tasks to an end
		  and how to change the topics
		*How to involve each child
		Cueing techniques
		Shaping techniques
		*Modelling techniques, esp.
		  for the teachers;
		  encouraging
		  teachers to use signs without
		  being directive
		* Makaton – knowing when to
		  apply signs, when to use
		  verbal language alone
		*Knowing when to respond
		  to a child's verbalisations
		  even when they are not in
		  intelligible
		*Responding to the
		  child's use signs
		* Knowing which children in
		  the group interact well,which
		  child can help to keep the
		  task moving
		* Involving passive children
		  in the activities
		*Directing the child's
		  attention using signs,
		  gestures, verbalisations,
		  physical prompts
		* Knowing when not to respond
		  to a child's verbalisation
		Selecting appropriate
		  materials for each child
		Managing child's behaviour

Psychological	Explaining skills
	Observation skills
	Interpersonal skills
	*Building the child's
	  self-confidence
		Monitoring skills
		Ongoing assessment/
		  observation of each child

Management	Planning and organising the therapy session	Time management
	Liaising with staff	Fitting in with the teacher(s)
	Recording/ongoing evaluation of each child's behaviour	Using a multidisciplinary approach
	Working as a team	

Therapist: A
Therapy: One-to-one adult with learning disability
Date: Jan. 91
Analysis: Recall without prompt and recall with prompt

Knowledge

Domain:	*Recall without prompt*	*Recall with prompt*
Speech and language	Level of linguistic ability Non-linguistic ability Non-verbal communication Pragmatics, use of signs, symbols	Knowledge of phonetics, phonology syntax, semantics, pragmatics Knowledge of how to analyse these long term effects of speech and language problems
Psychology	Level of literacy skills, level of attention, Level of cognitive ability *Personality traits	The acquisition of literacy skills Learning theories Behaviour modification techniques Lifestyles and their effects
Medical	Motor and visual difficulties *particularly regarding articulation skills General medical health and history	Sensory impairments Neurology Hearing problems Medical conditions associated with MH (Medical) expectations of adulthood
Policy	*Knowledge of the organisational structure of the day centre, staff etc. *Quality and standards of practice	Principles of normalisation Social attitudes to disability Social services provision
Assessment	Assessment of linguistic abilities Assessment of Makaton	Specific speech and language assessments Augmentative/alternative systems Assessment of the client's context Assessment of the client's likes and dislikes

| Management | Use of symbols, alternative systems; which signs to use, which to introduce, in what order etc.*
*Clinical evaluation: ongoing
Self evaluation: ongoing
Deciding when to intervene
*Positioning client correctly | Teaching functional communication
Alternative/augmentative techniques
Using a multidisciplinary approach
Personal awareness, professional development |

Skills

Domain:	Recall without prompt	Recall with prompt
Therapeutic/teaching	Varying order of presentation Awareness of the timing of presentation *Importance of positioning the client correctly *Maintaining client's interest Using appropriate vocabulary Using reinforcers *Facilitating conversation, not just 'Yes/No' responses! Assessing client's performance throughout session	Making a differential diagnosis Using appropriate assessments Programme planning Use of in-depth observation skills Investigate ways of changing the communication environment Structuring a learning situation Maintaining flexibility of presentation Establishing rapport Forming reciprocal relationships Using reinforcers appropriately Deciding on the correct timing of intervention Deciding on the correct timing of presentation Using vocabulary appropriately Respond to a wide range of verbal and non-verbal communication Cueing techniques Shaping techniques Carrying out a sequenced programme
Psychological	Listening skills Observation skills Explaining skills	Evaluating outcomes Explaining skills Assessing others' expectations Listening skills Observation skills Motivating others
Speech and language	Assessing client's communication throughout Appropriate use of symbols	Use of alternative/augmentative systems, e.g. signed communication
Management	Planning and organising the session Working as part of the team Self evaluation * 'Being prepared to say; I don't know!'	Goal planning Organisational skills Appointment making Helping client to make choices Maintaining/handling equipment

* Item not generated by consultative method

References

Abel, S. (1988) The mentally handicapped. In Rose, N. (ed.) *Essential Psychiatry* Oxford: Blackwell Scientific.

Abrahamson (1979) *Survey Methods in Community Medicine.* Edinburgh: Churchill Livingstone

Agar, M. (1980) *The Professional Stranger: an Informal Introduction to Ethnography.* London: Academic Press

American Speech Language Hearing Association (1990) *Demographic Profile of the ASHA Membership.* Washington: ASHA

Anderson, J. L. (1988) *Supervisory Processes in Speech Language Pathology.* Boston, MA: College Hill Press

Anderson, S.R. (1987) The management of staff behaviour in residential treatment facilities; a review of staff training techniques. in Hogg, J. and Mittler, P. (eds) *Staff Training in Mental Handicap.* London: Croom Helm

Anderson Levitt, K. M. and Platt, M. (1984) The speech of mentally retarded adults in contrasting settings. *UCLA Working Paper 28.* Los Angeles, CA: UCLA

Andrews, E. (1974) *The Emotionally Disturbed Family and Some Alternatives.* New York: Aronson

Argyle, M. (1975) *Bodily Communication.* London: Methuen

ASHA (1980) *Guidelines on the Employment and Utilization of Supportive Personnel.* ASHA March 1981. pp. 165–169

Atkinson, D. and Williams, F. (1990) *Know Me as I am: an Anthology of Prose, Poetry, and Art by People with Learning Difficulties.* London: Hodder and Stoughton

Austin, J.L. (1962) *How to Do Things with Words.* Oxford: Oxford University Press

Aylwin, S. (1988) In search of qualities: invited comments on Eastwood's qualitative research. *British Journal of Disorders of Communication* 23, 185–187

Bank-Mikkelsen, N. E. (1969) *Changing Patterns in Residential Services for the Mentally Retarded.* Washington DC: President's Committee on Mental Retardation

Barlow, D. H., Hayes, S. C. and Nelson, R. O. (1984) *The Scientist Practitioner: Research and Accountability in Clinical and Educational Settings.* Oxford: Pergamon Press

Barnes, S. (1988) The use of drama as a diagnostic tool with school aged language impaired children. *CSLT Bulletin 435*, 1–3

Barton, L. and Tomlinson, S. (1981) *Special Education: Policy, Practices and Social Issues.* London: Harper and Row

254

Bates, E. (1976) *Language in Context; the Acquisition of Pragmatics.* New York: Academic Press

Bates, E. and McWhinney B. (1982) The development of grammar. In Wanner, E. L. and Gleitman (eds) *Language Aquisition: the State of the Art.* Cambridge: Cambridge University Press

Bateson, G. (1972) *Steps to an Ecology of the Mind.* New York: Ballantyne Books

Beaumeister, A (1968) Behavioural inadequacy and variability in performance. *American Journal of Mental Deficiency* 73, 477–483

Beck, A. T. (1976) *Cognitive Therapy and the Emotional Disorders.* Philadelphia: Meridan

Bedrosian, J (1982) A sociolinguistic approach to communication skills; assessment and treatment methodology for mentally retarded adults. *Dissertation Abstracts International* 42, 4338A

Bedrosian, J. (1988) Adults who are mildly or moderately mentally retarded; communicative performance, assessment and intervention. In Calculator, S. and Bedrosian, J. (1988) *Communication Assessment and Intervention with Adults with Mental Retardation.* London: Taylor and Francis

Bedrosian, J. and Prutting, C.A. (1978) Communicative performance in mentally retarded adults in four conversational settings. *Journal of Speech and Hearing Research* 21, 79–95

Bench, R.J. (1989) Paradigm methods and the epistemology of speech pathology: some comments on Eastwood (1988). *British Journal of Disorders of Communication* 26, 235–242

Benson, B.A. Reiss, S. Smith, D.C. and Laman, D.S. (1985) Psychosocial correlates of depression in mentally retarded adults II: Poor social skills. *American Journal of Mental Deficiency* 89, 657–659

Bialystok, E. (1990) *Communication Strategies.* Oxford: Basil Blackwell

Blank, M., Gessner, M. and Esposito, A. (1979) Language without communication; a case study. *Journal of Child Language* 6, 329–52

Braddock, D. and Fujiura, G. (1991) Politics, public policy and the development of community services for the mentally retarded in the United States. *American Journal of Mental Retardation* 95, 369–387

Brandon, D. (1991) Peer advocacy and counselling. *Values into Action* 65, 8

Brechin, A. and Swain, J. (1986) *Shared Action Planning: a Skills Workbook in Mental Handicap Patterns for Living.* Milton Keynes: Open University Press

Brechin, A. and Swain, J. (1987) *Changing Relationships: Shared Action Planning with People with Mental Handicaps.* London: Harper and Row

Brechin, A. and Swain, J. (1988) Professional/client relationships; creating a working alliance with people with learning difficulties. *Disability, Handicap and Society* 3, 213–226

Brenneis, D. (1982) Making sense of settings; an ethnographic approach. *UCLA Working Paper 21.* Los Angeles, CA: UCLA

Brister, F. (1986) Incidence of occlusion due to impacted cerumen among mentally retarded adolescents. *American Journal of Mental Deficiency* 91, 302–304

Brown, L. et al. (1979) A strategy for developing chronological age appropriate and functional curricular content for severely handicapped adolescents and young adults. *Journal of Special Education* 13, 81–90

Brown, G. and Yule, G. (1983) *Discourse Analysis.* Cambridge: Cambridge Unversity Press

Brumfitt, S. (1985) Another side to therapy. *CLST Bulletin* 397 1–2

Brumfitt, S. and Clarke, P. (1983) An application of psychotherapeutic techniques to the management of aphasia. In Code, C. and Muller, D. (eds) *Aphasia Therapy.* London: Edward Arnold

Bryan, T.H. (1986) Self concept and attributions of the learning disabled. *Learning Disabilities Focus* 1, 82–89

Budd, S. (1981) Report on Speech Therapy Services for the Adult Mentally Handicapped in Nottinghamshire. Nottingham: Nottingham Health Authority

Bulpitt,D. and Turner, A. (1988) A joint approach; speech therapists and teachers working together. *CSLT Bulletin* 436, 5

Byng, S. (1988) Sentence Processing Deficits; theory and therapy. *Cognitive Neuropsychology* 5, 629–676

Byng, S. (1990) What is aphasia therapy? *Seventh Annual Mary Law Lecture for Action for Dysphasic Adults.* London: Royal Society of Medicine

Calculator, S. and Bedrosian, J. (1988) *Communication Assessment and Intervention with Adults with Mental Retardation.* London: Taylor and Francis

Cameron, L. Lester, R. and Lacey, B. (1988) Developing interaction and initiation skills in a group of adults with learning difficulties. *CLST Bulletin* 438, 3

Campaign for People with Mental Handicaps Annual Report 1986. London: CMH

Canadian Association of Speech Language Pathologists and Audiologists (1989) *CASLPA* November, p. 3–5.

Carrow, E. (1973). *Test for Auditory Comprehension of Language.* Windsor: NFER.

Caves, R. (1988) Consultative methods for extracting expert knowledge about professional competence. In Ellis, R. (ed) *Professional Competence and Quality Assurance in the Caring professions.* London: Croom Helm

Chaplin, K. and Turner, J. (1988) Intensive course initiaties change. *CST Bulletin* 435, 4–5

Chapman, R.S. (1972) A model of communication. University of Wisconsin: unpublished paper

Cheseldine, S. (1990) Book review of the Communication Assessment Profile (CASP). *British Journal of Disorders of Communication* 25, 260–261

Children Act (1990) London: HMSO

Chomsky, N. (1965) *Aspects of the Theory of Syntax.* Cambridge, MA: MIT Press

Clark, J.L. (1983) Language testing; past and present status – directions for the future. *Modern Language Journal* 67, 431–443

Cochrane, A. (1972) *Effectiveness and Efficiency.* London: Nuffield Hospitals Provincial Trust

Community Living (1990) What values are involved? *Community Living* 4, 2

Cook, T. and Campbell, D.T. (1979) *Quasi Experimentation.* Boston: Houghton Mifflin

Coolidge, F.L. Rakoff, R.J. Schellenbach, D. Bracken, D, and Walker, S. (1986) WAIS profiles in mentally retarded adults. *Journal of Mental Deficiency Research* 30, 15–17

Cottam, P. (1986) Speech therapy provision and management of mentally handicapped adults. *British Journal of Mental Subnormality* 32, 108–113

Coulter, A. (1991) Evaluating the outcomes of health care. In Gabe, J., Calnan, M. and Bury, N. (eds) *The Sociology of the Health Service.* London: Routledge

Cronbach (1975) Beyond the two disciplines of scientific psychology. *American Psychologist* 30, 116–127.

Crystal, D. (1969) *Prosodic Systems and Intonations in English.* Cambridge: Cambridge University Press

Crystal, D. (1982) *Profiling Linguistic Disability.* London: Edward Arnold

CSLT (1990) *Communications Quality; Professional Standards for Speech and*

Language Therapists. London: College of Speech and Language Therapists

Cullen, C. (1987) Nurse training and institutional constraints. In Hog, J. and Mittler, P. (eds) *Staffing Training in Mental Handicap*. London: Croom Helm

Cullen, C. (1988) A review of staff training: the emperor's old clothes. *Irish Journal of Psychology* 9, 309–323

Cullen, C. Burton, M. S., Watts, S. and Thomas, M. (1984) A preliminary report on the nature of interactions in a mental handicap institution. *Behaviour Research and Therapy* 21,579–583

Curtiss, S. (1977) *Genie: A Psycholinguistic Study of a Modern Day Wild Child*. New York: Academic Press

Curtiss, S., Kempler, D. and Yamada, J. E. (1981) The relationship between language and cognition in development. *UCLA Working Papers in Cognitive Linguistics* Volume 3. Los Angeles, CA: UCLA

Dalgliesh, M. (1983) Assessments of residential environments for mentally retarded adults in Britain. *Mental Retardation*. 21, 204–208

Davies, A. (1990) *Principles of Language Testing*. Oxford: Blackwell Scientific

Davies, P. (1979) *A Study of the Psychiatric and Psychological Assessment of Juveniles in the Child Care Services*. PhD dissertation, University of California, San Diego

Davies, P. and van der Gaag, A. (1992a) The professional competence of speech therapists. I Introduction and methodology. *Clinical Rehabilitation* 6, 209–214

Davies, P. and van der Gaag, A. (1992b) The professional competence of speech therapists. III. Skills and skill mix possibilities. *Clinical Rehabilitation* 6 311–324.

Davies, P. and van der Gaag, A. (1992c) The use and value of speech therapy assistants: introduction and methodology. Report to Department of Health.

Davies, P. and van der Gaag, A. (1992d) The use and value of speech therapy assistants II: an evaluation of process measures. *Clinical Rehabilitation* (in press)

Davies, P. van der Gaag, A. (1992e) The use and value of speech therapy assistants: summary and conclusions of a twelve month evaluation. *CSLT Bulletin* 494 (in press)

De Martino, M. (1954) Some characteristics of the manifest dream content of mental defectives. *Journal of Clinical Psychology* 10 175–8

Denmark, J. C. (1978) Early profound deafness and mental retardation. *British Journal of Mental Subnormality* 24, 81–89.

Department of Health (1989) *Working for Patients*. CM555, London: HMSO

Dewart, H. and Summers, S. (1989) *The Pragmatics Profile*. Windsor: NFER-Nelson

DHSS (1971) *Better Services for the Mentally Handicapped*. London: HMSO

DHSS (1980) *Mental Handicap: Progress, Problems and Priorities: A Review of Mental Handicap Services in England since the 1971 White Paper*. London: HMSO

DHSS (1981) *Care in the Community; a consultative document on moving resources for care in England*. London: HMSO

Dickens, P. (1983) *Guidelines on the Construction of Strengths and Needs Lists*. Unpublished manuscript, Stirling University

Dobson, S. (1990) *Report on Speech Therapy Services to Adults with Learning Difficulties*. Huddersfield Health Authority

Doll, G. (1985) *The Vineland Social Maturity Scales (Revised)*. Washington DC: American Guidance Service

Donabedian, A. (1980) *The Definition of Quality and Approaches to its Assessment*. Anne Arbor, MI: Health Administration Press

Dormandy, K. and van der Gaag, A. (1989) What colour are the alligators? A critical look at methods used to assess communication skills in adults with learning difficulties. *British Journal of Disorders of Communication* 24, 265–279

Dowson, S. (1991) Why isn't individual choice enough? *Values into Action* 65, 6–7

Dreeben, R. (1968) *On What is Learned in School.* New York: Addison Wesley

Dunn, L. M, and Dunn, L. M. (1982) *The British Picture Vocabulary Scales.* Windsor: NFER-Nelson

Eastwood, J. (1988) Qualitative research: an additional research methodology for speech pathology? *British Journal of Disorders of Communication* 23, 171–84

Edgerton, R. and Sabagh, G. (1962) From mortification to self aggrandizement: changing self conceptions in the careers of the mentally retarded. *Psychiatry* 25, 263–272.

Edgerton, R. (1963) A patient elite: ethnography in hospital for the mentally retarded. *American Journal of Mental Deficiency* 68, 372–85

Edgerton, R. (1967)*The Cloak of Competence; Stigma in the Lives of the Mentally Retarded.* Berkeley: UCLA Press

Edgerton, R. (1975) Issues relating to the quality of life among mentally retarded persons. In Begab, M. J. and Richardson, S. A. (eds) *The Mentally Retarded and Society: a Social Science Perspective.* Baltimore: UPP

Edgerton, R. (1984a) *Lives in Process; Mildly Retarded Adults Living in a Large City.* Washington: AAMR

Edgerton, R. (1984b) The participant observer approach in mental retardation. *American Journal of Mental Deficiency* 88, 498–505

Edgerton, R. and Bercovici, S. (1976) The cloak of competence; years later. *American Journal of Mental Deficiency* 80, 485–497

Edgerton, R. and Dingman, H. F. (1964) Good reasons for bad supervision: 'dating' in a hospital for the mentally retarded. *Psychiatric Quarterly Supplement* 38 221–233

Egan, G. (1984) People in systems: a comprehensive model for psychosocial education and training. In Larson, D. (ed.) *Teaching Psychological Skills.* Baltimore: Brookes Cole

Egan, G. (1990) *The Skilled Helper,* 4th edn. Baltimore: Brookes Cole

Elstob, L. (1986) Joint implementation – an intensive approach to adult training centre problems. *CST Bulletin* 416,1–2

Enderby, P. and Davies, P. (1989) Communication disorders: planning a service to meet the needs. *British Journal of Disorders of Communication* 24, 301–331

Enderby, P, Simpson, M. and Wheeler, P. (1992) *A Review of Therapy Services for Adults with Learning Difficulties in South West Regional Health Authority.* Report to SWRHA

Erickson, E. H. (1980) *Identity and the Life Cycle.* New York: Norton and Co

Errey, G. (1988) *ICAN Communicate.* London: Invalid Childrens Aid nationwide

Evans, G., Beyer, S. and Todd, S. (1987) *Evaluating the Impact of the All Wales Strategy on the Lives of People with a Mental Handicap.* Cardiff: Mental Handicap in Wales Applied Research Unit

Evans, G., Felce, D. and Hobbs (1991 *Evaluating Service Quality.* Standing conference on voluntary organisations, Cardiff

Fisher, S. (1983) Doctor–patient talk: how treatment decisions are negotiated in doctor–patient communication. In Fisher, S. and Todd, A. (eds) *The Social Organisation of Doctor Patient Communication.* Washington: Centre for Applied Linguistics

Florian, V. (1982) The meaning of work for physically disabled clients undergoing vocational rehabilitation. *International Journal of Rehabilitation Research* 5,

375–377.

Flynn, M. (1989) *Independent Living for Adults with Mental Handicap.* London: Cassell

Ford, J. (1985) Chaos: solving the unsolvable, predicting the unpredictable. In Barnsley, M. and Demko, S.G. (eds) *Chaotic Dynamics and Fractals.* New York: Academic Press

Fox, R. and Rotatori, A. (1982) Prevalence of obesity among mentally retarded adults. *American Journal of Mental Deficiency* 87,228–230

Fratelli, C. (1986) Are we reaching our goals? Developing outcome measures. In Larkins, P. (ed) *In Search of Quality Assurance: What Lies Ahead?* Washington: ASHA

Freeman, S. (1988) Giving mime a loud voice. *CLST Bulletin* 435, 3–4

Fromkin, V. and Rodman, R. (1978) *An Introduction to Language.* New York: Holt Rhinehart and Winston

Gazdar, G. (1979) Pragmatic constraints on linguistic production. In Butterworth, B. (ed.) *Language production,* Vol.1 London: Academic Press

General Clerical Test (1992) London: Harcourt Brace Jovanovich

Giddens, A. and Turner, J. (1987) *Social Theory Today.* Cambridge: Polity Press

Glaser, B.G. and Strauss, A.L. (1967) *The Discovery of Grounded Theory: Strategies for Qualitative Research.* Chicago: Adline

Glaser, R. and Nitko, A.J. (1971) *Measurement in learning and instruction.* In Thorndike, R.L. (ed) *Educaional Measurement.* Washington DC: American Council on Education

Gleick, J. (1987) *Chaos; Making a New Science.* London: Sphere Books

Goetz, J P. and Le Compte, M.D. (1984) *Characteristics and Origins of Educational Ethnography.* New York: Academic Press

Goffman, E. (1963) *Stigma; Notes on the Management of Spoiled Identity* Englewood Cliffs, NJ : Prentice Hall

Goffman, E. (1972) *Frame Analysis.* New York: Harper and Row

Goldenberg, I. and Goldenberg, H. (1980) *Family Therapy: An Overview.* Baltimore: Brookes Cole.

Goldstein (1990) Assessing clinical significance. In Olswang, L., Thompson, C., Warren, S. and Minghetti, N. (eds) *Treatment Efficacy Research in Communication Disorders.* Washington: ASHA

Goode, D. (1983) Who is Bobby? Ideology and method in the discovery of a Down's syndrome person's competence. In Keilhofner, D. (ed) *Health Through Occupation.* Philadelphia: FA Davis

Goode, D. (1984) Socially produced identities, intimacy and the problem of competence among the retarded. In Barton, L. and Tomlinson, S. (eds) *Special Education and Social Interests.* London: Croom Helm

Goodstein, H. A. (1982) The reliability of criterion referenced tests and special education. *Journal of Special Education* 16, 37–48

Graffam, J. (1983) About ostriches coming out of Communist China; meanings, functions and frequencies of typical interactions in group meetings for retarded adults. *UCLA Working Paper* 27 Los Angeles, CA: UCLA

Graffam, J. and Turner, J.L. (1984) Escape from boredom: the meaning of eventfulness in the lives of clients at a sheltered workshop. In Edgerton, R. (1984) *Lives in Process; Mildly Retarded Adults Living in a Large City.* Washington: AAMR

Green, R. (1991) A clinical supervision system in Riverside. *CSLT Bulletin* 470, 4

Green, R. (1992) Supervision as an essential part of practice. *Human Communication* 1, 21–22

Grice, H. (1975) Logic and conversation. In Code and Morgan (eds) *Syntax and Semantics.* Vol 3. New York: Academic Press

Griffiths, R. (1988) *Community Care; Agenda for Action: A Report to the Secretary of State for Social Services.* London: HMSO

Grunewald, K. (1971) *Menneskanipulering Pa Totalinstituioner; Fra Dehumanisering Til Normalisering.* Copenhagen, Denmark: Thaning and Appels Forlag

Grunwell, P. (1985) *Phonological Assessment of Child Speech (PACS).* Windsor: NFER-Nelson

Guess, D. (1984) Allowing the child greater participation in the educational process. Keynote address: Fifth Annual Montana Symposium, Early Education and the Exceptional Child. Billings, MT.

Gumperz, J. (1982) *Discourse Strategies.* Cambridge: Cambridge University Press

Gunzburg, H.C. (1963) *The Progress Assessment Chart.* Stratford: SEFA Publications

Guyette, T.W. (1978) A discussion of the use of the environmental approach to developing communication intervention programs with the mentally retarded. University of Kansas: Unpublished manuscript

Hallas, C. Fraser, W. and McGillivray, R. C. (1982) *The Care and Training of the Mentally Handicapped.* Edinburgh: J. Wright

Halle, J. (1988) Adopting the natural environment as the context of training. In Calculator, S. and Bedrosian, J. *Communication Assessment and Intervention for Adults with Mental Retardation.* London: Taylor and Francis

Halliday, M. (1970) *Learning How to Mean; Explorations in the Development of Language.* London: Edward Arnold

Halliday, M. (1978) *Language as Social Semiotic.* London: Edward Arnold

Halliday, M.A.K. and Hazan, R. (1976) *Cohesion in English.* London: Longman

Handy, C. (1975) *Understanding Organisations.* London: Penguin Educational

Hargreaves, D. (1978) What teaching does to teachers. *New Society* 43, 540–542

Harrell, C. (1990) Adapted techniques to improve hearing assessment. *Speech Therapy in Practice* 6, 7–8

Hawking, S. (1988) *A Brief History of Time.* London: Bantam Press

Haywood, H.C. and Switzky, H.N. (1985) Work responses of mildly mentally retarded adults to self versus external regulation as a function of motivational orientation. *American Journal of Mental Deficiency* 90, 151–159

Hermelin, B. and O'Connor, N. (1990) Factors and primes; a specific numerical ability. *Psychological Medicine* 20, 163–169

Hitchins, A. and Spence, R. (1991) *The Personal Communication Plan (PCP).* Windsor: NFER-Nelson

HMSO (1969) *Report of the Committee of Inquiry into Allegations of Ill Treatment of Patients and Other Irregularities at the Ely Hospital, Cardiff.* Cmnd 3975. London: HMOS

HMSO (1991) *Citizens' Charter.* London: HMSO

HMSO (1991) *Patients' Charter.* London: HMSO

Houts, P.S. and Scott, R.A. (1975) *Goal Planning with Developmentally Disabled People.* Pennsylvania State University

Howes, D. (1966) A word count of English. *Journal of Verbal Learning and Verbal Behaviour* 5, 572–604

Huberman, B. and Hogg, T. (1984) Understanding biological computation: reliable learning and recognition. *Proceedings of the National Academy of Sciences* 81, 6871–6875

Huddleston, R. (1984) *Introduction to the Grammar of English.* Cambridge: Cambridge Unversity Press

Humphreys, S., Lowe, K. and Blunden, R. (1984) *Long-Term Evaluation of Services for Mentally Handicapped People in Cardiff.* Cardiff: Mental Handicap in Wales Applied Research Unit

Hurst Brown, L. and Keens, A. (1990) *ENABLE: Encouraging a Natural and Better Life Experience.* London: Forum Consultancy

Hymes, D. (1971) Competence and performance in linguistic theory. In Huxley, R. and Ingram, E. (eds) *Language Acquisition: Models and Methods.* London: Academic Press, p.3–28

Hymes, D. (1974) *Foundations in Sociolinguistics.* Philadelphia: University of Pennsylvania Press

Illsley, R. (1980) *Professional Medicine or Public Health.* Oxford: Blackwell Scientific

Ingham, J. C. (1990) Issues in treatment efficacy. In Olswang, L., Thompson, C., Warren, S. and Minghetti, N. (eds) *Treatment Efficacy Research in Communication Disorders.* Washington: ASHA

Inglehart, R.F. and Woodward, M (1972) Language conflicts and political community. In Giglioli, P. *Language and Social Context.* Harmondsworth: Penguin

Ingram, D. E. (1985) Assessing proficiency: an overview on some aspects of testing. In Hytanstam, K. and Pienemann, M. (eds) *Modelling and Assessing Second Language Acquisition.* Clevedon: Multilingual Matters

Jackendoff, R. (1972) *Sematic Interpretation in Generative Grammar.* Cambridge Mass: MIT Press

Jackendoff, R. (1983) *Semantics and Cognition.* Cambridge, MA: MIT Press

Jacobs, M. (1990) *Psycho-dynamic Counselling in Action.* London: Sage

James, W. (1890) *The Principles of Psychology.* New York: Holt Rhinehaut Winston

Jay Report (1979) *Report to the Committee of Enquiry into Mental Handicap Nursing and Care.* Cmnd 7468. London: HMSO

Jeffree, D. and Cheseldine, S. (1986) *Pathways to Independence.* Kidderminster: BIMH

Jones, J., Tuner, J. and Heard, A. (1992) Making Communication a Priority. *CSLT Bulletin* **478**, 6–7

Jones, S. (1990) *INTECOM: A Package Designed to Integrate Carers into Assessing and Developing the Communication Skills of People with Learning Difficulties.* Windsor: NFER-Nelson

Jussim, L. (1986) Self fulfilling prophesies: a theoretical and integrative review. *Psychological Review* **93**, 429–445

Kagan, N. (1984) Interpersonal process recall in Larson, D. (ed) *Teaching Psychological Skills.* Baltimore: Brookes Cole

Kaufman, S. (1984) Friendship, coping systems and community adjustment of mildly retarded adults. In Edgerton, R. *Lives in Process; Mildly Retarded Adults Living in a Large City.* Washington: AAMR

Kelly, O. J. and McReynolds, L. (1988) Clinical perceptions of the role of research in the clinic. University of Kansas: Unpublished manuscript

Kent, R. D. (1989) The fragmentation of clinical service and clinical science in communicative disorders. *National Student Speech Language Hearing Association Journal* **17**, 4–16

Kernan, K. T. and Turner, J. L. (1986) It's just a dream: the use of dream narratives by the mentally retarded. *UCLA Working Paper* 36. Los Angeles, CA: UCLA

Kernan, K. T. and Sabsay, S. (1989) Communication in social interactions: aspects of an ethnography of communication of mildly mentally handicapped adults. In Beveridge, M., Conti-Ramsden, G. and Leudar, I. (eds) *Language and*

Communication in Mentally Handicapped People. London: Chapman and Hall

Kersner, M. (1987) Working with the mentally handicapped through drama. *CSLT Bulletin* **422** 1–2

Kersner, M. (1988) *Ali Baba and the Forty Thieves; a Play*. London: Alphabet Books

Kersner, M. (1988) *A Space Oddity; a Play*. London: Alphabet Books

Kersner, M. (1992) *Tests of Voice Speech and Language*. London: Whurr Publishers

Kiernan, C,. and Jones, M. (1982) *The Behaviour Assessment Battery*. Windsor: NFER-Nelson

King, K. D., Raynes, N. V., and Tizard, J. (1971) *Patterns of Residential Care: Sociological Studies in Institutions for Handicapped Children*. London: Routledge Kegan Paul

Kings Fund (1984) *Advocacy Project* Paper 51. London: King's Fund

King's Fund (1980) *An Ordinary Life*. Project Paper 24. London: King's Fund

King's Fund (1988) *Ties and Connections: An Ordinary Community Life for People with Learning Difficulties*. London: King's Fund

Klein, R. (1991) *Health Care Provision under Financial Constraint; a Decade of Change*. London: Royal Society of Medicine

Koegel, P. (1978) The creation of incompetence; socialisation and mildy retarded persons. *UCLA Working Paper 6*. Los Angeles, CA: UCLA

Kropka, B. and Williams, C. (1986) The epidemiology of hearing impairment in people with mental handicap. In Ellis, D. (ed.) *Sensory Impairments in Mentally Handicapped People*. London: Croom Helm

Kuhn, T. S. (1970) *The Stucture of Scientific Revolutions*. Chicago: University of Chicago Press

Laban, R. (1951) The educational and therapeutic value of the dance. In *The Dance has Many Faces*. New York: World Press

Lanarkshire Social Services (1985) *Report on Day Services for Mentally Handicapped Adults*. Lanark: Lanarkshire Social Services

Landesman, Dwyer, S. and Knowles, M. (1987) Ecological analysis of staff training in residential settings. In Mittler, P. and Hogg, J. (eds) *Staff Training in Mental Handicap*. London: Croom Helm

Langer, E. J. (1983) *The Psychology of Control*. London: Sage

Language Testing (1984) London: Edward Arnold

Leech, G. (1971) *Meaning and the English Verb*. London: Longman

Leech, G. (1983) *Principles of Pragmatics*. London: Longman

Leudar, I. (1989) Communication environments for mentally handicapped people. In Beveridge, M., Conti Ramsden, G. and Leudar, I. (eds) *Language and Communication in Mentally Handicapped People*. New York: Chapman Hall

Leudar, I. and Fraser, W. (1985) How to keep quiet; some withdrawal strategies in mentally handicapped adults. *Journal of Mental Deficiency Research* **29**, 315–30

Levinson, C. (1983) *Pragmatics*. Cambridge: Cambridge University Press

Levitt, G. (ed) (1987) *The Creative Tree*. Salisbury: Michael Russell

Levy, P. (1988) Further comments on Eastwood's 'qualitative research'. *British Journal of Disorders of Communication* **23**, 189

Linder, S. (1978) Language context and the evaluation of the verbal competence of the mentally retarded. *UCLA Working Paper* **1**. Los Angeles, CA: UCLA

Lorenz, J. 1963 Deterministic nonperiodic flow. *Journal of the Atmospheric Sciences* **20**, 448–464

Lyle, J.G. (1960) Some factors affecting the speech dvelopment of imbecile children in an institution. *Journal of Child Psychology and Psychiatry* **1**, 129–129

Lyons, J. (1977) *Semantics 1.* Cambridge: Cambridge University Press

McBrien, J. (1981) Introducing the EDY Project. *Special Education: Forward Trends* **8**, 29–30

McCartney, E., Kellet, B. and Warner, J. (1984) Speech therapy provision for mentally handicapped people: the results of a preliminary survey. *CST Bulletin* **384**, 1–3

MacDonald, J. (1985) Language through conversation. In Warren, S.F., Rogers, C. and Warren, A.K. (eds) *Teaching Functional Language: Generalisation and Maintenance of Language Skills.* Baltimore: UPP

McIntyre, B. (1981) Drama as an adjunct to speech therapy for children. In Schattner, G. and Courtney, R. (eds) *Drama in Therapy.* New York: Drama Book Specialist

McLaren, J. and Bryson, S. (1987) Review of recent epidemiological studies of mental retardation; prevalence, associated disorders and etiology. *American Journal of Mental Retardation* **92**, 243–254

McQueen, D.M. Peskin, C. (1983) Computer assisted design of pivoting disc prosthetic mitral valves. *Journal of Thoracic and Cardiovascular Surgery* **86**, 126–135

McQueen, P., Spence, M., Garner, J., Pereira, L. and Winsor, E. (1987) Prevalence of major mental retardation and associated disabilities in the Canadian Maritime Provinces. *American Journal of Mental Deficiency* **91**,460–466

McReynolds, L. (1990) Historical perspectives of treatment efficacy research. In Olswang, L., Thompson, C., Warren, S. and Minghetti, N. (eds) *Treatment Efficacy Research in Communication Disorders.* Washington: ASHA

McTear, M. (1985) Pragmatic disorders: a case study of conversational ability. *British Journal of Disorders of Communication* **20**, 129–142

Manpower Planning Advisory Group (MPAG) (1990) *Speech Therapy: An Examination of Staffing Issues.* London: MPAG

Martin, J.P. (1984) *Hospitals in Trouble.* Oxford: Blackwell Scientific

Masilover, M. and Knowles, J. (1982) *The Derbyshire Language Scales.* Derbyshire County Council

Medawar, P. (1982) *Plato's Republic.* Oxford: Oxford University Press

Mehan, H. (1979) *Learning Lessons.* Cambridge MA: Harvard University Press

Merrill, E.C. (1985) Differences in semantic processing speed of mentally retarded and non retarded persons. *American Journal of Mental Deficiency* **90**, 71–80

Miles, J. (1984) Strange attractors in fluid dynamics. *Advances in Applied Mechanics* **24**, 189–214

Miller, C. (1990) The music behind the words. *CSLT Bulletin* **454**, 2–3

Miller, E. and Gwynne, G. (1972) *A Life Apart.* London: Tavistock Publications

Miller, J. (1978) Assessing childrens' language behaviour: a developmental process approach. In Schiefelbusch, R.L. (ed.) *Bases of Language Intervention*, Volume 1. Baltimore: UPP

Minifie, F. (1983) ASHA – from adolescence onwards. *ASHA* **17**, 17–21

Mittler, P. (1984) Evaluation of services and staff training. In Dobbing, J. (ed) *Scientific Studies in Mental Retardation.* London: Macmillan

Morris, P. (1969) *Put Away.* London: Routledge and Kegan Paul

Morse, J. (1988) Assessment procedures for people with mental retardation; the dilemma and suggested adaptive procedures. In Calculator, S. and Bedrosian, J. (eds) *Communication Assessment and Intervention with Adults with Mental Retardation.*London: Taylor and Francis

Murphy, J. (1987) Assessment and therapy with adults. *Speech Therapy in Practice*. 3, 30–32

Naglieri, J. A. (1985) Assessment of mentally retarded chidlren with the Kauffman Assessment Battery for children. *American Journal of Mental Deficiency*. 89, 367–371

National Council for Vocational Qualifications (1988) *Introducing National Vocational Qualifications; Implications for Education and Training*. London: NCVQ

National Development Group (1978) *Services for Mentally Handicapped People in Hampshire*. London: National Development Group

National Development Group (1984) *National Development Group Fourth Report 1981–1984*. London: HMSO

National Development Team for Mentally Handicapped People (1976) *Mental Handicap: Planning Together no 1*. London: NDT

National Development Team for Mentally Handicapped People (1985) Fourth Report. London: NDT

Neisser, U. (1967) *Cognitive Psychology*. New York: Appleton-Century-Crofts

Nihira, K., Foster, R., Shellhaas, M. and Leland, H. (1975) *The Adaptive Behaviour Scales*. Washington: AAMR

Nirje, B (1969) The normalisation principle and its human management implications. In Kugel, R. and Wolfensberger, W. (eds) *Changing Patterns in Residential Services for the Mentally Retarded*. Washington DC: Presidents' Commitee on Mental Retardation

Noble, A. (1990) *A Survey of the Speech Therapy Needs of Adults Attending a Resource and Activity Centre*. Bath: Health Authority

Nolan, M., McCartney, E., McArthur, K., and Rowson, V. J. (1980) A study of the hearing and receptive vocabulary of trainees in an adult training centre. *Journal of Mental Deficiency Research*. 24, 271–286

Normand, C. (1991) *Clinical Audit in Professions Allied to Medicine and Related Therapy Professions*. Queen's University, Belfast: Health and Health Care Research Unit

Normansfield Hospital (1978) *Report to the Committee of Enquiry into Normansfield Hospital*. London: HMSO

North, M. (1972) *Personality Assessment Through Movement*. Plymouth Books

O'Brien, J. and Tyne, A. (1981) *The Principle of Normalisation: A Foundation for Effective Services*. London:CMH

Ochs, E. (1979) Social foundations of language. In Freddle, R. (ed) *New Directions in Discourse Processing, Vol.3*, pp.207–221. Norwood NJ: Ablex

O'Connor, N. (1989) The performance of the idiot savant: implicit and explicit.*British J Disorders of Communication*. 24, 1–21

O'Connor, N. and Hermelin, B. (1987) Visual and graphic abilities of the idiot savant artist. *Psychological Medicine*. 17, 79–90.

Oller, J. W., and Kahn, F. (1981) Is there a global factor of language proficiency? In Read, J. A. S. (ed.) *Directions in Language Testing*. Singapore University Press, 3–39

Olswang, L. (1990) Treatment efficacy research: a path to quality assurance. In Olswang, L., Thompson, C., Warren, S., and Minghetti, N. *Treatment Efficacy Research in Communication Disorders* Washington: ASHA

Oswin, M. (1978) *Children in Long Stay Hospitals*. London: Spastics International Medical Publications

Owings, N. and Guyette, T. W. (1982) Communication behaviour assessment and treatment with the adult retarded: an approach. *Speech and Language:*

Advances in Basic Research and Practice 7,185–216.

Owings, N. and McManus, M. (1980) An analysis of communicative functions in the speech of a deinstitutionalised mentally retarded client. *Mental Retardation* **18**, 309–314.

Owings, N., McManus, M., and Scherer, N. (1981) A deinstitutionalised retarded adult's use of communication functions in a natural setting. *British Journal of Disorders of Communication* **16**, 119–128

Palmer, F. (1965) *A Linguistic Study of the English Verb*. London: Longman

Palmer, W. and Dawson, P. (1992) *Self Advocacy at Work*. Nottingham: EMFEC

Parker, M., and Liddle, K. (1987) The communication needs of the mentally handicapped population in west Berkshire – a survey. *CLST Bulletin* **428**, 1–2

Parry, G. and Watts, F. (1989) *Behavioural and Mental Health Research: a Handbook of Skills and Methods*. London: Lawrence Earlbaum Associates

Peters, T. J,. and Waterman, R. H. (1982) *In Search of Excellence*. London: Harper and Row

Pfeffer, N. and Coote, A. (1991) *Is Quality Good for You? A Critical Review of Quality Assurance in Welfare Services*. London: Institute of Republic Policy Research

Pickering, M. (1987) Supervision: a person focused process. In Crago, J. and Pickering, M. (eds) *Supervision in Human Communication Disorders: Perspectives on a Process*. Boston: College Hill Press

Pickering, M. (1988) Interpersonal communication and the supervisory process; the search for Ariadne's thread. In Anderson, J. L. (1988) *Supervisory Processes in Speech Language Pathology*. Boston, MA: College Hill Press

Pickett, J. and Flynn, P. T. (1983) Language assessment tools for mentally handicapped adults; survey and recommendations. *Mental Retardation* **21**, 244–247

Pinney, S. and Ferris Taylor, R. (1989) Breaking down the barriers. *Speech Therapy in Practice* **5**, 4–6

Pirie, M. (ed.) (1991) *Empowerment*. London: Adam Smith Institute

Planck, M. (1949) *Scientific Autobiography and Other Papers*. Translated by F. Gaylor

Planck, M. (1900) quoted in Heisenberg, W. Born, M., Schrodinger, E,. and Ayer, P. (1961) *On Modern Physics*. New York: Clarkston N Potter

Platt, M. (1985) Displaying competence: peer interaction in a group home for retarded adults. *UCLA Working Paper 29*. Los Angeles, CA: UCLA

Pletts, M. (1981) Principles and practice of clinical teaching – a need for structure. *British Journal of Disorders of Communication* **16**,129–134

Popham, W. (1981) *Modern Educational Measurement*. New York: Prentice Hall

Price Williams, D. and Sabsay, S. (1979) Communicative competence among severely retarded persons. *Semiotica* **26**, 35–63

Prutting, C.A. and Kirchner, D.M. (1983) Applied pragmatics. In Gallagher, T. and Prutting, C. (eds) *Pragmatic Assessment and Intervention Issues in Language*. San Diego: College Hill Press.

Puddicombe, B. (1991) *Days; Challenge to Consensus* series. London: VIA. Publications

Purkiss, A. and Hodson, P. (1982) *Housing and Community Care*. National Council for Voluntary Organisations. London: Croom Helm

Reiter, S. and Levi, A.M. (1980) Factors affecting social integration of noninstitutionalised mentally retarded adults. *American Journal of Mental Deficiency* **85**, 25–30

Richardson, SA. and Ritchie, J. (1989) *Developing Friendships: Enabling People with Learning Difficulties to make and maintain Friends*. London: Policy Studies Institute

Rogers, C. (1951) *Client Centred Therapy*. Boston: Houghton Mifflin

Rondal, J. and Lambert, J. (1983) The speech of mentally retarded adults in a dyadic communication situation; some formal and informative aspects. *Psychologica Belgica* 23, 49–56

Rose, G. (1991) What is supervision? *CSLT Bulletin* 470,5–6

Rosen, A. and Proctor, E. (1981) Distinctions between treatment outcomes and their implications for treatment evaluation. *Journal of Consulting and Clinical Psychology* 49,418–425

Rotatori, A., Switzky, H. and Fox, R. (1983) Obesity in mentally retarded, psychiatric and non handicapped individuals: a learning and biological disability. In Gadow, K. and Bailer, I. (eds) *Advances in Learning and Behavioural Disabilities*, Vol 2. Greenwich, CT: JAI Press

Rowan, S. (1990) *Speech Therapy in Practice*.

Royal National Institute for the Deaf (1990) Fair Hearing Campaign

Ryan, B. (1971) Operant procedures applied to stuttering therapy for children. *Journal of Speech and Hearing Disorders* 36, 264–280

Ryan, B. and van Kirk, B. (1974) The establishment, transfer and maintenance of fluent speech in 50 stutterers using delayed auditory feedback and operant procedures. *Journal of Speech and Hearing Disorders* 39, 3–10

Ryan, J. Thomas, F. (1987) *The Politics of Mental Handicap*. London: Free Association Books

Sabsay, S. and Platt, M. (1984) Weaving the cloak of competence. *UCLA Working Paper 32*. Los Angeles, CA: UCLA

Sacks, H., Schegloff, E. and Jefferson, J. (1974) A simplest systematics for the organisation of turntaking for conversation. *Language* 50, 696–675

Sarno, M.T., (1969) *The Functional Communication Profile*. New York: University Medical Centre

Savignon, S. (1985) Evaluation of Communicative Competence. *Modern Language Journal* 69, 129–134

Schaffer, W.M. and Kot, M. (1985) Nearly one dimensional dynamics in an epidemic. *Journal of Theoretical Biology* 112, 403–427

Scott, J., Ross, A. and van der Gaag, A. (1987) The changing role of speech therapists who work wth adults who have mental handicaps. *CST Bulletin* 424, 15

Scott, M. and Marinker, M. (1992) Imposed change in general practice. *British Medical Journal* 304, 1548–1550

Scott, M. L. and Madsen, H. (1983) The influence of re-testing on test affect. In Oller, J.W. (ed) *Issues in Language Testing Research*. Rowley, MA: Newbury House

Searle, J. (1969) *Speech Acts*. Cambridge: Cambridge University Press

Searle, J.R. (1976) The classification of illucutionary acts. *Language and Society* 5, 1–24

Seigel, G. and Spradlin, J. (1985) Therapy and research. *Journal of Speech and Hearing Disorders* 50, 226–230

Shackleton Bailey, M. (1983) *The Hampshire Assessment for Living with Others*. Hampshire Social Services

Shearer, A. (1976) The news media. In Kugel, R. and Shearer, A. (eds) *Changing Patterns of Residential Services for the Mentally Handicapped*. Washington: Presidents' Committee for the Mentally Retarded

Shenton, J. (1990) Dance Movement and Mental Handicap. *Therapy Weekly* 22 November

Sherbourne, V. (1971) 'Explorations' (video available from Concord Films Council,

210 Felixstowe Rd Ipswich, Suffolk)

Shohamy, E. (1983) Inter-rater and intra-rater reliability of the oral interview and concurrent validity with cloze procedures in Hebrew. In Oller, J. W. Jr. (ed) *Issues in Language testing Research.* Rowley MA: Newbury House

Sines, D.T. (1985) *The Role and Function of the Community Nurse for People with a Mental Handicap.* Report of a Working Party of the RCN Community Mental Handicap Nurses Forum. London: Royal College of Nursing

Sinha, C. (1986) Psychology, education and the ghost of Kasper Hauser. *Disability, Handicap and Society* 1, 245–259

Skinner, B.F. (1938) *The Behaviour of Organisms.* New York: Appleton Century Crofts

Skinner, C., Wirz, S., Thompson, J. and Davidson, J. (1984) *The Edinburgh Functional Communication Profile.* Windsor: NFER-Nelson

Smith, D.S., Godenberg, E., Ashburn, A., Kinsella, G., Sheikh, K., Brennan, P.J., Meade, T., Zutshi, D., Perry, J. and Reeback, J. (1978) Remedial therapy after stroke. *British Medical Journal* 282,517–520

Social Services Inspectorate (1989) *Inspection of Day Services for People with a Mental Handicap.* London: Department of Health

Sollenberger, H. (1978) Development of correct use of the FSI oral interview. In Clark, J.L.D. (ed) *Direct Testing of Speaking Proficiency: Theory and Application.*

Sperber, D. and Wilson, D. (1986) *Relevance.* Oxford: Blackwell Scientific

Stange, W. (1980) AMICI Theatre Company, London

Stansfield, J. (1982) Current trends in speech therapy with mentally handicapped people. *CSLT Bulletin* 365, 1–2

Sternlicht, M. (1966) Dreaming in adolescent institutionalised mental retardates. *Psychiatric Quarterly* 10, 97–99

Strong, C. (1991) Jigsaw Theatre Company, Glasgow

Swartz, S. (1977) *Naming, Necessity and Natural Kinds.* Cornell University Press

Tallal, P. (1988) Developmental language disorders. In Kavanaugh, J. and Truss, T. (eds) *Learning Disabilities; Proceedings of the National Conference.* Parkton, MD: York Press

Taylor, J. and Taylor, K. (1986) *Mental Handicap: Partnership in the Community?* London: Office of Health Economics

Terrell, G. (1991) Hearing aid use in adults with learning difficulties. *College of Speech and Language Therapists Bulletin* 470, 2–3

Tew, B. (1979) The Cocktail Party syndrome in children with hydrocephalus and spina bifida. *British Journal of Disorders of Communication* 14, 89–102

Todd, A. (1983) A diagnosis of doctor–patient discourse in the prescription of contraception. In Fisher, S. and Todd, A. (eds) *The Social Organisation of Doctor–Patient Communication.* Washington: Centre for Applied Linguistics

Tomlinson, R. (1982) *Disability Theatre and Education.* London: Souvenir Press

Townsend, P. (1969) Foreword. In Morris, P. (ed.) *Put Away.* London: Routledge Kegan Paul

Turner, J.L. (1982) Workshop society: ethnographic observations in a work setting for retarded adults. *UCLA Working Paper 20.* Los Angeles, CA: UCLA

Turner, J., Kernan, K. and Gelphman, S. (1984) Speech etiquette in sheltered Workshop. In Edgerton, E. (ed) *Lives in Process.* Washington: AAMR

Tyler, L. and Wessels, J. (1983) Quantifying contextual contributions to word recognition processes. *Perception and Psychophysics* 34, 409–420

Tyne, A. (1978) *Looking at Life in Hospital, Hostel, Home or Unit.* London: Campaign for the Mentally Handicapped

van der Gaag, A. (1985) *The Effects of Social Environment on the Word Associations of the Mentally Handicapped.* MSc thesis.

van der Gaag, A. (1987) The development of a language and communication assessment procedure for use with adults with a mental handicap – an interim report. *British Journal of Mental Subnormality* **34**, 62–68

van der Gaag, A. (1988) *The Communication Assessment Profile (CASP).* London: Speech Profiles

van der Gaag, A. (1989a) Joint assessment of communication skills: formalising the role of the carer. *British Journal of Mental Subnormality* **35**, 22–28

van der Gaag, A. (1989b) The view from Walter's window: social environment and the communicative competence of adults with a mental handicap. *Journal of Mental Deficiency Research* **33**, 221–227

van der Gaag, A. and Davies, P. (1992a) The professional competence of speech therapists. II knowledge base. *Clinical Rehabilitation* **6**, 215–224

van der Gaag, A. and Davies, P. (1992b) The professional competence of speech therapists IV Attitude and attribute base. *Clinical Rehabilitation* **6**, 325–332

van der Gaag, A. and Davies, P. (1992c) The use and value of speech therapy assistants III: an evaluation of service users and service providers, perceptions. *Clinical Rehabilitation* (in press)

van der Gaag, A. and Davies, P. (1992d) The use and value of speech therapy assistants V: training and supervision issues. *Human Communication* **2**, 16–18

van der Gaag, A. and Davies, P. (1992e) The use and value of speech therapy assistants VI: who are they and what do they do? *Human Communication* **2**, 20–23

van der Gaag, A. and Davies, P. (1993) Following the dolphins: an ethnographic investigation of speech and language therapists. *European Journal of Disorders of Communication*, in press

van der Gaag, A. and Lawler, C. (1990) The validation of a language and communication assessment procedure for use with adults with learning difficulties. *Scottish Office Health Bulletin,* September

Vanier, J. (1982) *The Challenge of L'Arche.* London: Darton, Longman and Todd

Values into Action (1991) The Calderdale Campaign. *Values into Action* **63**, 6–7

Vogel, S. (1987) Dialogues with the mentally handicapped: the effect of type of interaction and audience on conversation. University of Manchester: MSc thesis

Vygotsky, L. (1986) *Thought and Language.* Cambridge MA: MIT Press

Walsh, W. (1920) Dreams of the feeble minded. *Medical Record* **97**, 395–398

Ward, L. (ed) (1986) *Getting Better All the Time? Issues and Strategies for ensuring Quality in Services for People with Mental Handicap.* University of Bristol, Department of Mental Health

Ward, L. (1988) Whose home is it anyway? *Community Care* 14 Jan

Warnock, M. (1979) *Report to the Committee of Enquiry into the Education of Handicapped Chidren and Young People.*Cmnd 7212 London: HMSO

Warren, S,. Rogers, Warren, A. K., Baer, D. and Guess, D. (1980) Assessment and facilitation of language generalisation. In Sailor, W., Wilcox, B., and Brown, L. *Methods of Instruction for Severely Handicapped Students.* Baltimore: Paul Brookes

Watson, J. B. (1919) *Psychology from the Standpoint of a Behaviourist.* Philadelphia: Lippincott

Weir, R. (1962) *Language in the Crib.* The Hague: Mouton

Welsh Office (1983) *The All Wales Strategy for the Development of Services for Mentally Handicapped People.* Cardiff: Welsh Office

Wesche, M. B. (1983) Communicative testing in a second language. *Modern Language Journal* 67, 1–55

West, R. and Ansberry, M. (1968) *The Rehabilitation of Speech.* New York: Harper and Row

Whelan, E., and Speake, B. (1977) *Adult Training Centre Services in England and Wales–Report of the First National Survey.* London: National Association of Teachers of the Mentally Handicapped

Whelan, E., and Speake, B. (1979) The Copewell Assessment Chart. Kidderminster: BIMH

Whewell, W. (1847) *The Philosophy of the Inductive Sciences*

Whitefoot, S. and Tuck, L. (1990) *Discovering Communication: A Course Outline*

Wiess, R. S. (1975) *Loneliness: The Experience of Emotional and Social Isolation.* Cambridge MA: MIT Press

Williamson, G. (1991) An ethnography of communication within an Adult Training Centre for people with learning difficulties. Open University: MSc thesis

Wilson, D. N. (1979) When is a team not a team? An observation of community mental handicap teams. *Apex* 7, 94

Wilson, M. and Evans, M. (1980) *Education of Disturbed Pupils.* London: Schools Council

Wolf, A. (1983) Simplicity and universality in the transition to chaos. *Nature* 305, 182

Wolfensberger, W. (1972) *The Principle of Normalisation in Human Services.* Toronto: National Institute on Mental Retardation

Wolfensberger, W. (1983) Social role valorisation: a proposed new term for the principle of normalisation. *Mental Retardation* 21, 234–39

Wolfensberger, W. (1980) Overview of normalisation. In Flynn, J. and Nitsch, K. (eds) *Normalisation, Social Integration and Community Services.* Baltimore: University Park Press

Wolfensberger, W. (1988) Common assets of mentally retarded people that are not commonly acknowledged. *Mental Retardation* 26, 63–70

Wootton, G. (1992) Exploring the client–therapist relationship in dysphasia. *Human Communication.* 1, 20–21

Yeates, S. (1980) *The Development of Hearing: Its Progress and Problems.* Studies in Developmental Paediatrics, Vol 2. Lancaster: MIT Press

Yeates, S. (1989) Hearing in people with mental handicaps. A review of 100 adults. *Mental Handicap.* 17, 33–37

Zetlin, A. G. and Sabsay, S. (1980) Characteristics of verbal interaction among moderately retarded peers; some methodological issues. *UCLA Working Paper 13*

Zetlin, A. G, and Turner, J. L. (1984) Self perspectives in being handicapped: stigma and adjustment. In Edgerton, R. (1984) *Lives in Process; Mildly Retarded Adults Living in a Large City.* Washington: AAMR

Zigler, E. (1961) Social deprivation and rigidity in the performance of feeble minded children. *Journal of Abnormal and Social Psychology* 62, 413–21

Zigler, E. and Balla, D. A. (1972) Developmental course of responsiveness to social reinforcement in normal children and institutionalised retarded children. *Developmental Psychology* 6, 66–73

Index